Clinical Guide to Bioweapons and Chemical Agents

W0091052

Vincent E. Friedewald

Clinical Guide to Bioweapons and Chemical Agents

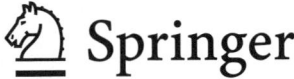 Springer

Vincent E. Friedewald, MD
University of Notre Dame
Notre Dame, Indiana

ISBN: 978-1-84628-255-3   e-ISBN: 978-1-84628-787-9
DOI: 10.1007/978-1-84628-787-9

British Library Cataloguing in Publication Data
Friedewald, Vincent
    Clinical guide to bioweapons and chemical agents
    1. Communicable diseases – diagnosis   2. Poisons   3. Symptoms
    4. Emergency medicine – Diagnosis   5. Bioterrorism – Health aspects   6. Chem-
    ical terrorism – Health aspects   I. Title
    616′.075
    ISBN-13: 9781846282553

Library of Congress Control Number: 2007928824

Printed on acid-free paper

9 8 7 6 5 4 3 2 1

Springer Science+Business Media
springer.com

To my loving wife, Julie, and our precious family,
Natalie, Vincent III, and Jake

About the Author

Dr. Friedewald is a graduate of the University of Notre Dame (BS) and the University of Texas Southwestern Medical School (MD). He completed his residency in internal medicine and cardiovascular diseases at Baylor College of Medicine in Houston, Texas. He is Board-certified in Internal Medicine and Cardiology.

For over 25 years, Dr. Friedewald practiced internal medicine and cardiology, initially in 1971 as Director of Diagnostic Laboratories at the Arizona Heart Institute in Phoenix. In 1976 he assumed the position of Chief of Cardiology and Chairman of the Department of Internal Medicine at the Honolulu Medical Group at Queen's Medical Center in Honolulu. He returned to Houston in 1982 to practice cardiology as a member of the faculty at Baylor and serve as Director of the Cardiac Noninvasive Laboratory and the Cardiac Rehabilitation Program at the Kelsey-Seybold Clinic.

His initial medical research was in the development of echocardiography, which was the basis for his *The Textbook of Echocardiography*, and computer-based analysis of cardiac monitoring systems, including electrocardiography, exercise testing, and vectorcardiography. In recent years, he has focused on studies of the evolutionary role of informational media and the impact of electronic media on human behavior; electronic publishing; voice recognition technology medical applications; and medication adherence by patients.

Dr. Friedewald has faculty appointments at the University of Notre Dame (Research Professor, College of Science and Senior Research Fellow in Ethics) and the University of Texas Health Sciences Center at Houston (Clinical Professor of Internal Medicine). He is Assistant Editor of *The American Journal of Cardiology*.

Since February, 2002, Dr. Friedewald has been Medical Director of Argus1, a Web-based program for the early detection of biological and chemical attack and other naturally-occurring and accidental public health threats. Argus1 is used for point-of-care decision support by physicians, physicians' assistants, nurses, first responders (police, fire, emergency medical specialists), in hospital emergency departments, medical clinics, school clinics, health departments, and other institutions and agencies responsible for individual and community health.

Foreword

When I began collaborating with the author's father, Vincent Friedewald, Sr. in the early 1980s, I could not have imagined the form that this project would eventually take. The project we collaborated on – developing a computerized approach to medical diagnosis – was already hugely innovative for its time. As personal computers began to come into popular use, Friedewald, Sr. envisioned a software program that would enable physicians to key in patient symptoms and get back an accurate diagnosis. The program that he helped develop, called *Med-Diatec*, was tested at the Baylor College of Medicine, where I was then serving as Chair of the Department of Medicine. It was an exciting project to work on, right at the dawn of the computer age, before anyone knew to what extent computer technology would become integrated into our daily lives. What made the project even more remarkable was how far it had progressed from its previous incarnation. Long before computers were to enter homes and offices, in 1953 Friedewald, Sr. patented a cleverly designed system of interlocking index cards, each containing various symptoms and signs to aid the physician in the diagnostic process.

More than five decades later, his son, Vincent Friedewald, Jr., has compiled an authoritative guide for general practitioners and clinicians in the event of a bioterrorist attack or public health crisis. Inspired by his father's visionary work and drawn from the original computer database of diseases and symptoms, this book by Friedewald, Jr. is an invaluable resource. Systematically organized according to infections and poisons, complications, and bodily systems, it is designed to facilitate prompt, efficient responses in the event of an emergency. After the unfortunate events of September 11, 2001, our world changed in ways that no one could have foreseen. Like his father before him, Vincent Friedewald, Jr. has created a resource that is both a testament to the past and a handbook for the future.

Antonio M. Gotto, Jr., MD, DPhil
The Stephen and Suzanne Weiss Dean
and Provost for Medical Affairs
Weill Cornell Medical College

Preface

Tularemia and the First Medical Computer

The first medical computer was invented in 1944 by my father, Vincent Friedwald, Sr., MD <http://www.argus1.com/?medicalcomputer> (Figure 1).

While studying for internal medicine board examinations during service in the United Sates Navy in World War II, it struck my dad that standard textbooks had limited value in the patient care setting, because they were organized according to diseases – not by patient symptoms or physical findings, which are the starting point for every diagnosis. He translated key diagnostic data of each condition onto 3- × 5-inch white index cards, 1 card for each disease. As the stack of cards grew, he envisioned a machine (Figure 2) which, through an intricate construction of holes punched in the cards (Figures 3–6), would provide differential diagnoses according to matching symptoms, signs, and other diagnostic information keyed into the machine. After discharge from the military, he pursued his dream of a medical diagnosis machine while practicing internal medicine in the small West Texas town of Big Spring. In 1948 he applied for patent protection of the machine – *the first medical computer*. The sample disease in the patent application was Tularemia (Figure 3), which he had researched as a student at St. Louis University Medical School in the mid-1930s. Tularemia would be 1 of 5 conditions to be classified as category "A" biological weapons in a new threat to civilization 50 years after the patent application.

On May 12, 1953, he was awarded Patent number 2,638,215 by the U.S. Patent Office for a "Card Sorting Mechanism" (Figure 7). Like many dreams, however, his vision of a medical computer would lay dormant – but not forever.

In 1980, unable to continue active medical practice due to disability from the disease polymyalgia rheumatica, he resurrected his dream. He shared the index cards – stored in faded cardboard shoe boxes for almost 30 years – with Mr. Robert Burns, a pioneer

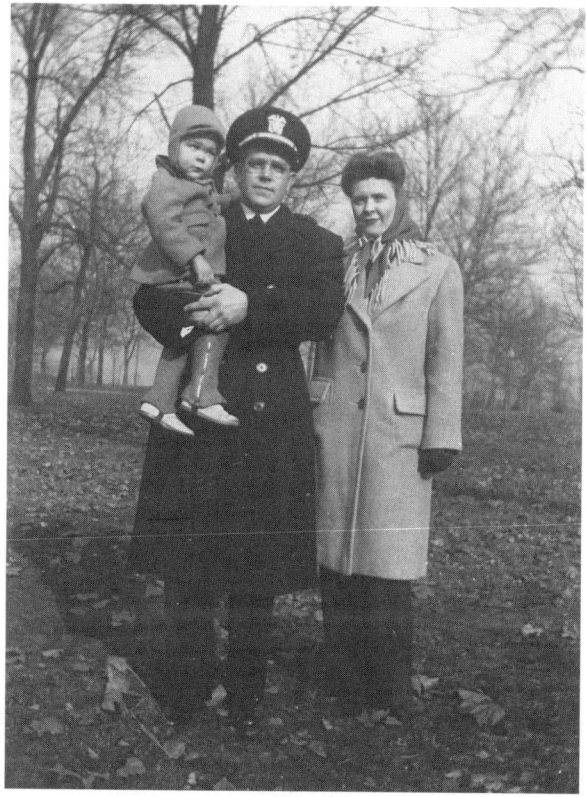

Figure 1. Dr. Vincent Friedewald, Sr., with his wife, Eleanor, and their son, Vincent Jr., the author.

specialist in medical information technology in Houston, and together they converted the original database of over 800 diseases and 1,000 signs and symptoms into a software program named *Med-Diatec* ("Medical Diagnostic Technology"). He also collaborated with Dr. Antonio Gotto, then Chair of the Department of Medicine at Baylor College of Medicine, and several other members of the faculty at Baylor to expand and test the database.

On September 10, 1990, with his medical computer at last a working reality, he and my mother, Eleanor – his ardent supporter for over 50 years – passed away.

(*Continued on page xix*)

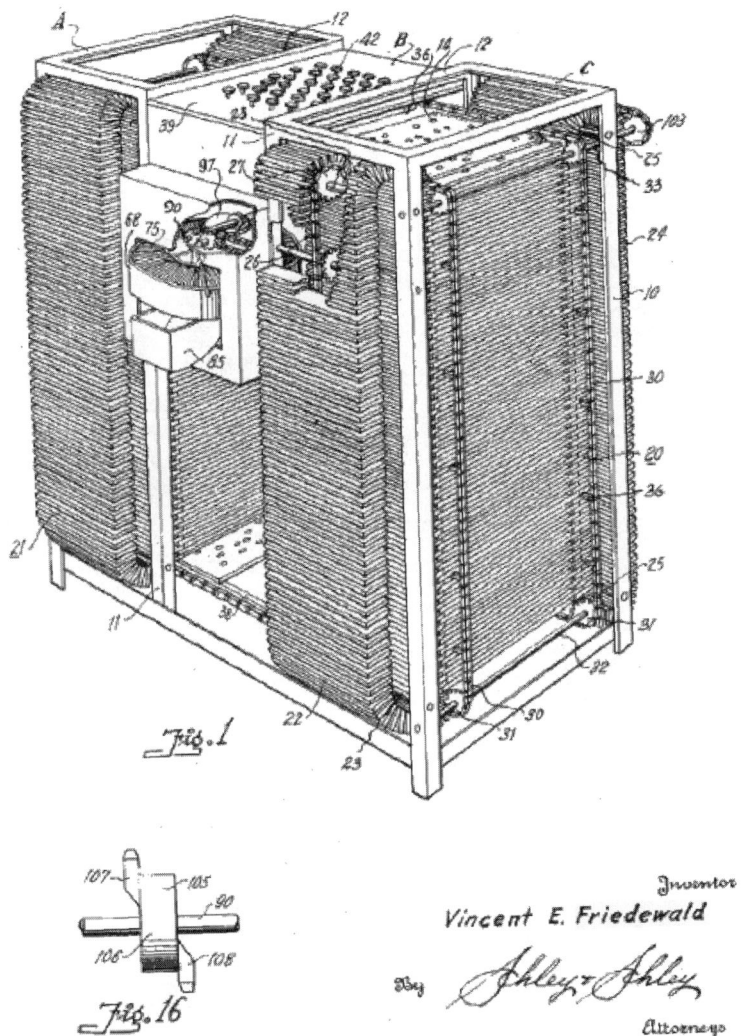

Figure 2. The first medical computer: diagnostic card-sorting machine designed by Dr. Friedewald, Sr.

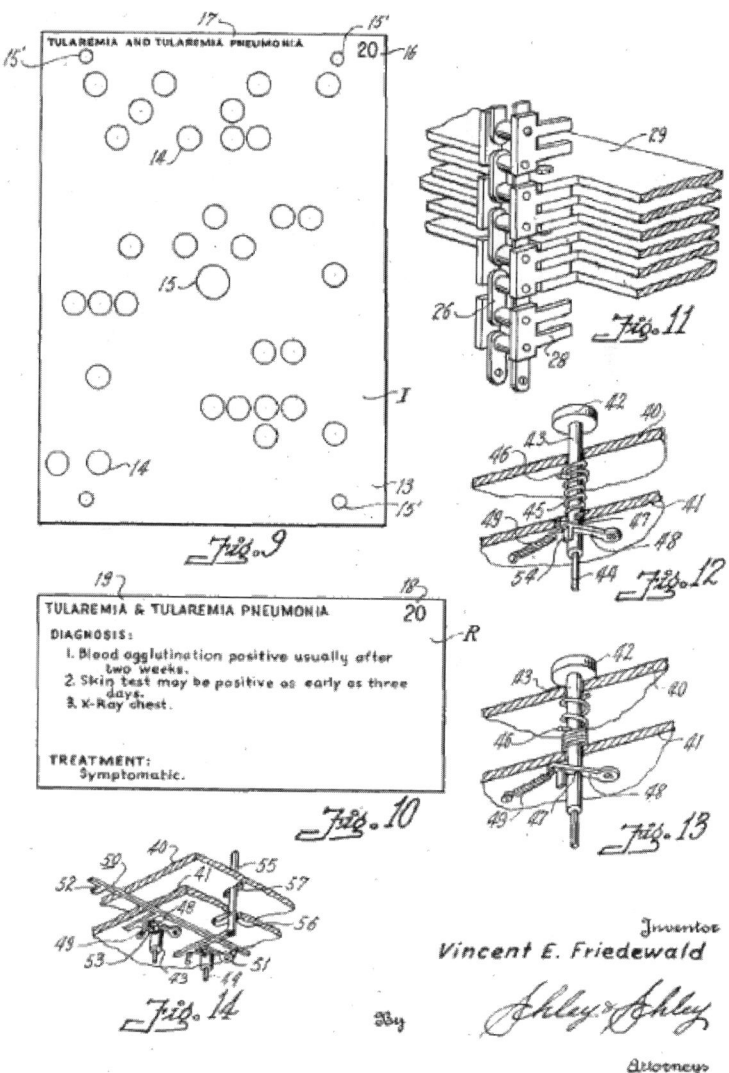

Figure 3. Punch-holed disease plate for card-sorting machine. Note that the disease sample for the patent application is "TULAREMIA AND TULAREMIA PNEUMONIA," how a Category A weapon of bioterrorism.

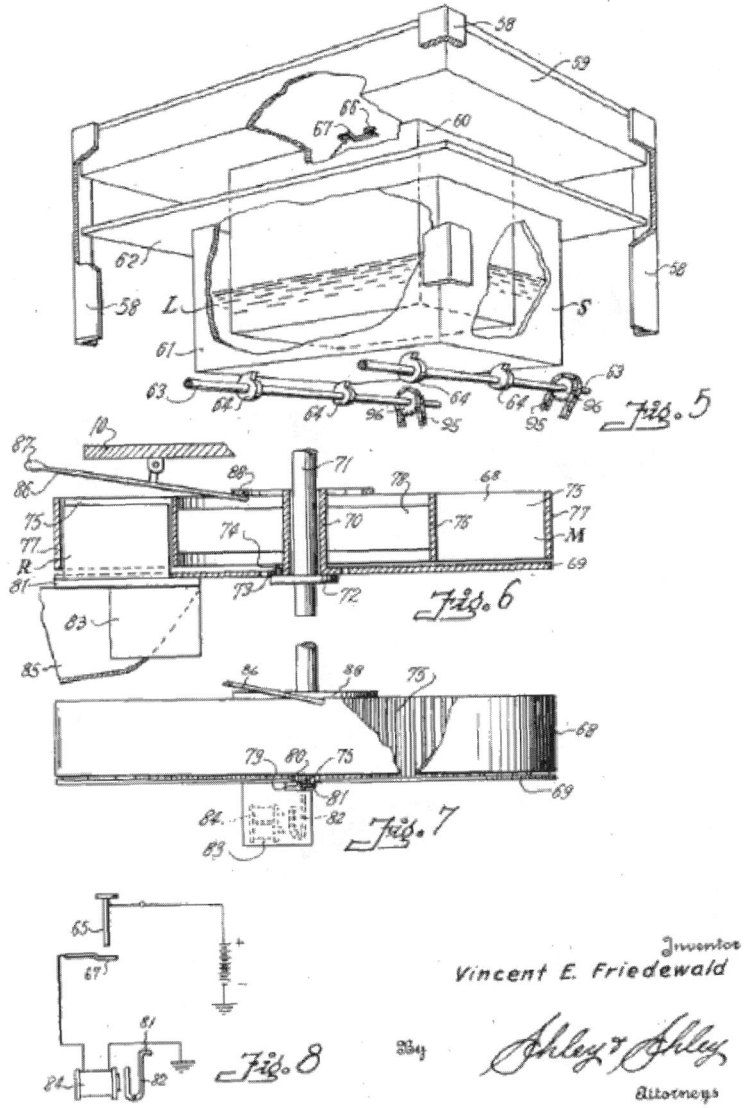

Figure 4. Punch hole design.

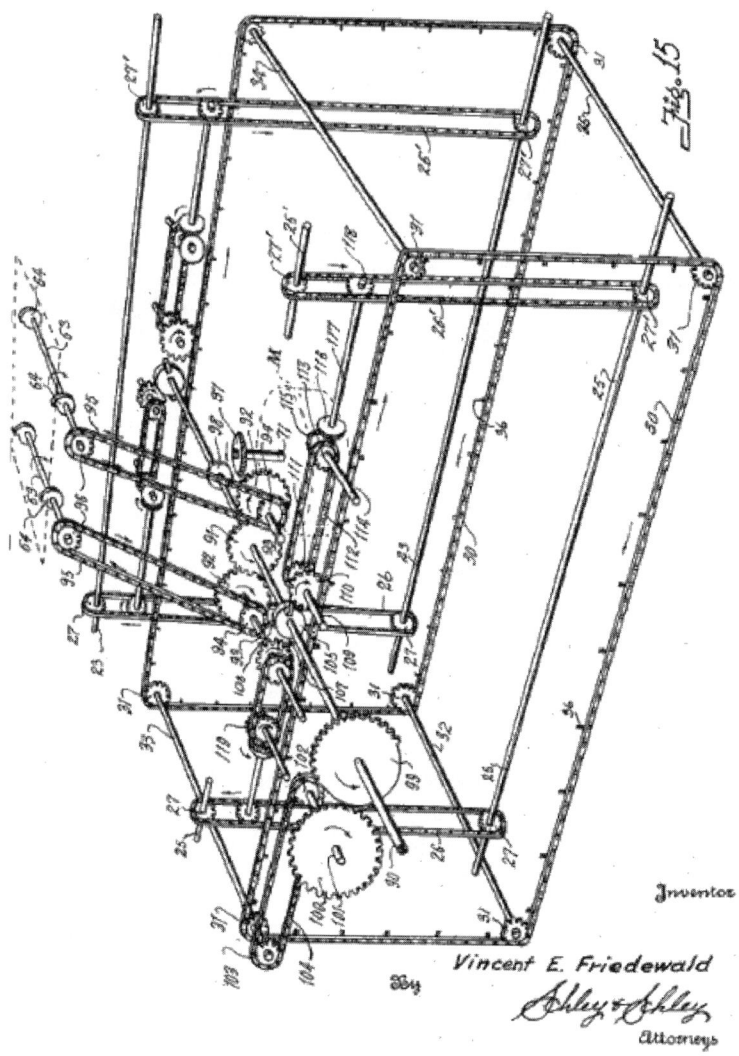

Figure 5. Cog system.

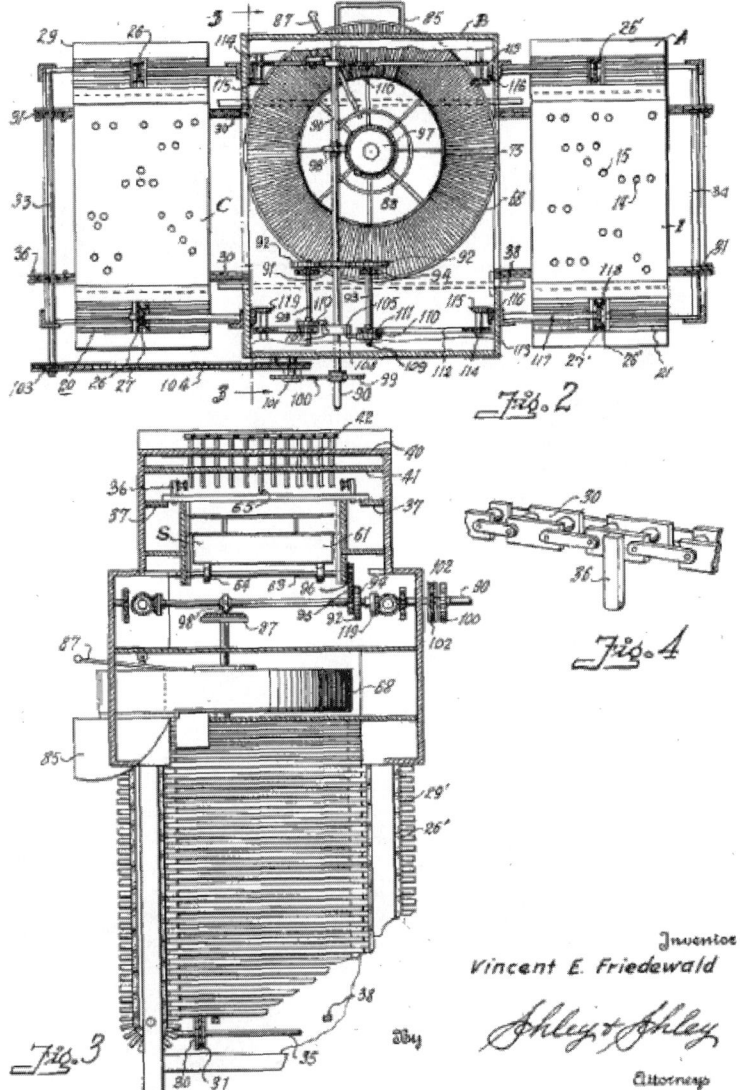

Figure 6. Card-sorting mechanism.

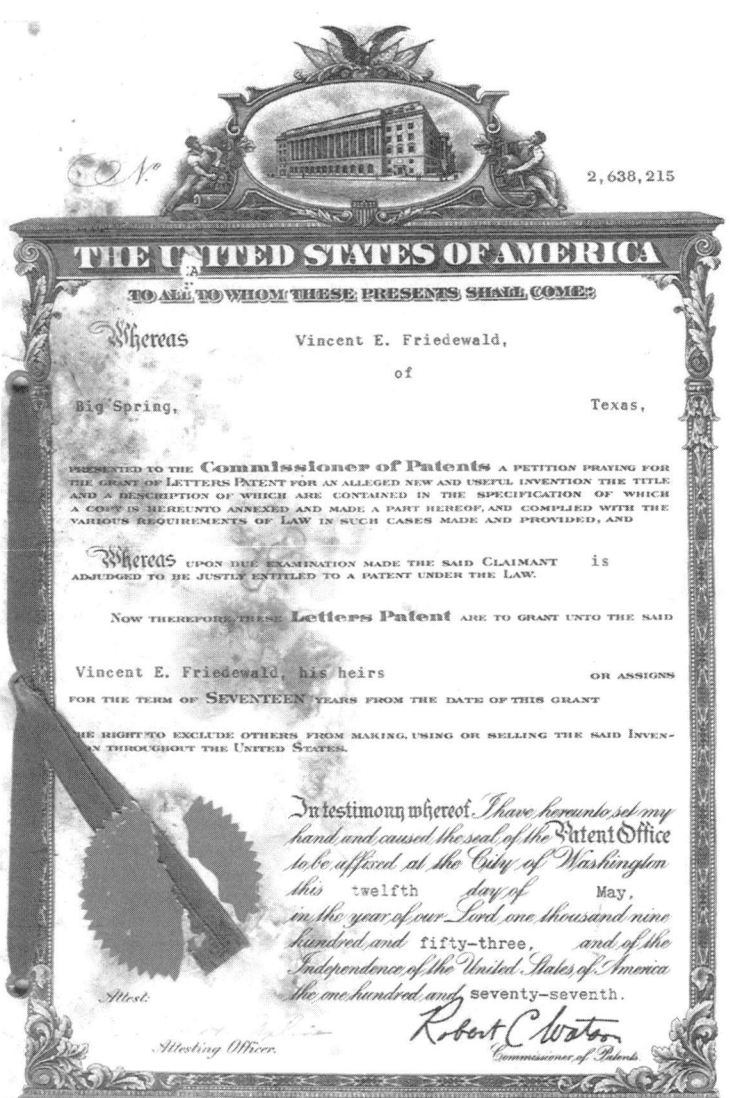

Figure 7. Cover of patent award number 2,638,215 to Dr. Friedwald, Sr, May 12, 1953.

My dad's original machine is now a Web-based software program, *Argus1* – named for the Greek god of surveillance – for point-of-care diagnosis and disease management. The *Clinical Guide to Bioweapons and Chemical Agents* is derived from the Argus1 database, which had its beginning on index cards in 1944 somewhere in a jungle or swamp during a war most of us know only from history books. The *Clinical Guide* is written for healthcare specialists' use in pandemics, select disease outbreaks, and another war we pray will never happen.

Vincent E. Friedewald

Contents

Section Two
Clinical Guide—Poisons **279**

Using the *Guide*

The *Clinical Guide to Bioweapons and Chemical Agents* is a point-of-care reference for the diagnosis and initial treatment of selected infectious agents and poisons that have been transmitted intentionally (biological, chemical, or radiation terrorism), by accident, or as part of natural public health outbreaks.

The *Guide* format is mainly comprised of key words and phrases, making it usable at the patient point-of-care, where rapid retrieval of information is important. The format throughout is consistent, and the content is targeted at information relevant to patient management in the setting of emergent clinical care.

The Conditions

There are 3 classes of conditions in the *Guide*:

Section 1. Infections: conditions listed in the United States Centers for Disease Control (CDC) *Emergency Preparedness and Response: Bioterrorism Agents/Diseases.* In addition, many public health diseases are included that may require differentiation from terrorist biological events, such as Avian Influenza, Chickenpox and West Nile Fever.

Section 2. Poisons: conditions listed in the United States Centers for Disease Control *Chemical Emergencies.*

Section 3. Complications: acute, often life-threatening conditions that occur secondary to infections and poisonings. A patient can present for care for the first time with the complication of a condition, which can add to the difficulty in making the primary diagnosis. Only relevant diagnostic information is provided because specific treatment varies according to the primary etiologic agent.

Sections 1 and 2 – Infections and Poisons

There are 23 sections in each Infection and Poison.

Weapon

"No" states that the condition has not been labeled as a possible terrorist agent, but may require differentiation from a bioweapon.

CDC Bioterrorism Category: _

Category A: high-priority agents include organisms that pose a threat to national security because they:

- can be easily disseminated or transmitted from person to person
- result in high mortality rates and have the potential for major public health impact
- might cause public panic and social disruption
- require special action for public health preparedness

Category B: second highest priority agents include those that:

- are moderately easy to disseminate
- result in moderate morbidity rates and low mortality rates
- require specific enhancements of CDC's diagnostic capacity and enhanced disease surveillance

Category C: emerging pathogens that could be engineered for mass dissemination in the future because of:

- availability
- ease of production and dissemination
- potential for high morbidity and mortality rates and major public health impact

CDC Hazardous Chemical Category: _

Designation of hazardous chemicals that may be used as terrorist weapons:

- Biotoxins
- Blister agents/vesicants
- Blood agents
- Choking/lung/pulmonary agents

- Incapacitating agents
- Long-acting anticoagulants
- Metals
- Nerve agents
- Organic solvents
- Radiation
- Toxic alcohols

Alternate Names: other names, which differ among geographical areas sometimes confusing disease identification and reporting.

Example (Bolivian Hemorrhagic Fever):
>Black typhus
>Machupo virus
>South American hemorrhargic fever

Etiology: the infectious or chemical agent. When known and relevant to clinical understanding, a brief description of the disease process is also described.

Example (Anthrax):
>Bacillus anthracis

>Spores germinate to bacillary form, multiply in macrophages, release toxins causing edema, hemorrhage, and tissue nerosis; tissue damage caused by release of toxins – protective antigen, lethal toxin, edema toxin

Transmission

"Source": natural or military origins of the agent.

"Entry": means of agent entry into the body (inhalation, ingestion, contact, bite, injection).

"Human-to-Human": whether transmission of the condition can occur directly from one human to another human ("Yes" or "No") without an intervening vector.

Example (Q Fever):

Source:	Infected dust and other materials from many animals, including sheep, cattle, goats, rodents, ticks
Entry:	Contact Inhalation
Human-to-Human:	Rare

Predisposing/Comorbid Conditions: preexisting diseases and other factors that increase the likelihood of contracting the condition and/or may cause a more serious clinical course.

Example (Influenza):
> Chronic obstructive pulmonary disease
> Heart disease
> Third-trimester pregnancy

Demographics

"Locations": where the condition naturally occurs. "Global" means all geographical areas are vulnerable.

"Populations": persons especially prone to contract the condition with accidental (poisons) or natural (infections) transmission. "All" means that all population groups are vulnerable.

"Calendar": time of year the condition naturally exists or peaks. "Year-round" means there is no predilection for time of natural occurrence.

Example (Rift Valley Fever):

Location:	Africa, Arabian peninsula
Populations:	Livestock workers, veterinarians, anyone exposed to mosquitoes in endemic area
Calendar:	Year-round

Systems: body anatomical or physiological systems *mainly* affected by the condition. Most conditions of the severity used in terrorist attacks, however, affect multiple systems, and the systems listed *should not be regarded as restrictive*; rather, these lists should be used *only* as general guides to aid in rapid diagnosis.

Example (Ebola Hemorrhagic Fever):
        Coagulation
        Gastrointestinal
        Nervous
        Optic
        Skin

Incubation (Infections) or Time to Clinical Onset (Poisons): usual time interval from exposure to the infection or chemical until the *first* onset of symptoms.

Example (Lassa Fever):
        1-3 WEEKS

Signs/Symptoms: physical findings (signs) and complaints (symptoms). The anatomical or physiological part of the body is to the left of the hyphen and the abnormality is to the right of the hyphen.

Example: "Chest, ant – pain, pleuritic"

Medical terms for abnormalities are in parentheses.

Example: "Eyes, pupils – dilation (mydriasis)"

Differentiation: select conditions that are clinically similar. *This list is not intended to be complete*, and varies with time of year, geographic location, and other concurrent diseases in the community.

Example (Tularemia):
Includes, but not limited to:
        Atypical pneumonia
        Bacterial pneumonia
        Influenza
        Other causes of infectious
           lymphadenopathy and
           dermopathy
        Q fever

Complications: conditions that may occur secondarily. Diagnostic features of some complications are described in the chapter, "Complications". *This list is not intended to be complete.*

> Example (Cholera):
> *Include, but not limited to:*
> > Hypoglycemia
> > Hypovolemic shock
> > Metabolic acidosis
> > Noncardiac pulmonary edema
> > Pneumonia
> > Renal failure
> > Sepsis
> > Spontaneous abortion

Laboratory: tests that *may* be abnormal and are usually performed in clinical laboratories or available from specialized laboratories. The test sample and item measured is to the left of the hyphen, the abnormality on the right of the hyphen, and the medical term is in parenthesis. Test results greatly vary among patients, and interpretation must be made only in the overall clinical context of each case.

> Example: "Blood WBC – increased (leukocytosis)"

ECG: electrocardiographic abnormalities, if any.

> Example: "ST segment – depressed"

Imaging: abnormalities that may be detected by radiography, magnetic resonance imaging, computed tomography, ultra-sound, or other imaging modalities.

> Example: Lungs, parenchyma – nodule, solitary

Other Tests: specialized tests performed when a specific diagnosis is considered.

> Example: Liver biopsy – granulomas, inflammation

Treatment – Nonpharmacologic: non-drug therapies. Details such as frequency and duration are variable and are beyond the scope of the *Guide*. Readers should refer to current treatment guidelines and to the *Clinical Guide* Web site for links to specific conditions.

> Example (Dengue):
> > Fluids and electrolytes
> > Fresh plasma
> > Oxygen
> > Plasma expanders

Treatment – Pharmacologic: generic drug therapies. Details such as frequency and duration are variable and are beyond the scope of the *Guide*. Readers should refer to current treatment guidelines and to the *Clinical Guide* Web site for links to specific conditions.

> Example (Q Fever):
> > Antibiotics
> > > Chloramphenicol
> > > Quinolones
> > > Rifampin
> > > Tetracycline

Treatment – Surgical/Invasive: treatments using invasive procedures.

> Example (Radiation Poisoning):
> > Bone marrow transplant
> > Burn care

Precautions: select strategies to protect first-responders and other caregivers, who should refer to current guidelines for further details, as this list is not all-inclusive.

> Example (Phosgene Poisoning):
> > Protective clothing: yes
> > Site decontamination: yes
> > Other: SCBA

Primary Prevention: select strategies for prevention in vulnerable populations. Readers should refer to current guidelines for additional strategies, as this list is not all-inclusive.

Example (Plague):
>   Vaccine: yes
>   Animal reservoir control
>   Environmental control
>   Post-exposure antibiotic prophylaxis
>   Avoid travel to endemic/epidemic areas or take
>   appropriate precautions when doing so

Course: usual patient outcomes, with and without treatment, and mortality.

Example (Anthrax):

Untreated
>   Cutaneous – 20% fatal
>   Gastrointestinal – 25–60% fatal
>   Inhalational – 100% fatal

Treated
>   Cutaneous – mortality
>   Gastrointestinal – unknown
>   Inhalational – 60% cured in post 9-11 cases, but much
>   higher mortality in prior series of natural outbreaks

Notes: bracketed numbers in all sections are referenced here, with additional information about specific items that may be useful in diagnosis and treatment.

Example (Smallpox):
>   [14]   May occur on palms and soles, which is unusual
>   in chickenpox

▲ This symbol denotes a special threat to patients, emergency responders, laboratory personnel, or caregivers.

☠ This symbol denotes an item relating to mortality.

Updates

A Web address (URL) unique to each condition is displayed. Readers are encouraged to go to this Web site to view timely updates on conditions in the *Guide*.

Example: (Lassa Fever)
"http://www.argusl.com/?lassa"
The general directory site is "http://www.argusl.com/?home"

Section 3—Acute Complications

This section provides signs and symbols of selected complications of the conditions in Sections 1 and 2, and key tests that may aid in their diagnoses.

Limitations of the *Guide*

1. Reporting methodologies vary and some entities have been much better studied than others. Thus, the clinical findings of some conditions in the *Guide* are likely incomplete.
2. Many of the conditions are rarely – if ever – seen outside of relatively small geographic areas among restricted populations. Exactly how these conditions would be clinically manifest if they occurred in other larger and distant populations with different genetic codes, diets, and environments is speculative.
3. Agents disseminated as weapons might present unique diagnostic and treatment challenges from the same naturally-transmitted conditions. (For example, the anthrax event in the USA in 2001 involved a child < 1 year of age, the first such reported infection in that age group)
4. There are probably more – yet to be identified – infections and poisonings that could be used as terrorist weapons than are in the *Guide*.

CLINICAL GUIDE—INFECTIONS

Anthrax

Weapon
CDC Bioterrorism Category: A

Alternate Names [20]
Cutaneous anthrax [C]
Gastrointestinal anthrax [G]
Inhalational anthrax [I]
Woolsorter's disease [I]

Etiology
Bacillus anthracis [6]

Spores germinate to bacillary form, multiply in macrophages, release toxins causing edema, hemorrhage, and tissue necrosis; tissue damage caused by release of toxins – protective antigen, lethal toxin, edema toxin [29]

Transmission
Source:	Spores from infected animals, esp cattle and sheep
Entry:	Contact [C]
	Inhalation [I]
	Ingestion [G]
Human-to-Human:	No

Predisposing/Comorbid Conditions
Open skin lesion [C]
Lung disease [I]

Demographics
Location:	Global
Populations:	All [31]
Calendar:	Year-round

Systems

Gastrointestinal
Lymphatic
Musculoskeletal
Nervous
Oropharynx
Respiratory – lower
Skin

Incubation

Cutaneous: 1-12 days
Gastrointestinal: Indeterminate
Inhalation: 1-60 days

Signs/Symptoms [17, 24]

Abdomen, RLQ – mass [34]
Abdomen – fluid (ascites) [G]
Abdomen – pain [1]
Appetite – reduced (anorexia)
Bowel movements – blood or black (melena) [G]
Bowel movements – diarrhea [G]
Breathing – difficult, rest (rest dyspnea) [I]
Breathing – rapid (tachypnea) [I]
Breath sounds, basilar – decreased
Breath sounds – crackling (rales) [I]
Chest, ant – pain, pleuritic [1]
Chest, local – percussion dullness [I]
Chest – pain, pleuritic [I]
Chills
Cough – nonproductive [I]
Cough – productive [16]
Extremities, upper unilat – edema [21]
Face – edema [C] [14]
Fatigue
Head – pain (headache)
Heart rate – rapid (tachycardia) [15]
Joints – pain (arthralgia)
Lymph nodes, regional – enlarged [2]
Lymph nodes, gen – enlarged
Mentation – confusion

Mentation – weakness (malaise)
Mood – lethargy
Mouth, mucosa – edema [G]
Mouth – ulcers [G]
Muscles – pain (myalgia)
Muscles – weak
Nausea
Neck, post – stiff (meningismus)
Nose – drainage (rhinorrhea, coryza) [23]
Skin, single lesion – draining [C]
Skin, single lesion – edematous [C] [12, 13]
Skin, single lesion – red (erythematous) [C]
Skin, single lesion – itching, burning [C] [11]
Skin, single lesion – macule/papule [C] [8]
Skin, single lesion – necrosis [C] [3]
Skin, single lesion – ulcer [C]
Skin, single lesion – vesicle [C]
Skin color, local – red (erythema) [C]
Speech, voice – hoarse [G]
Swallowing – difficult (dysphagia) [G]
Sweating – night
Sweating – increased (hyperhydrosis)
Temperature, body – elevated (fever) [22]
Throat – edema [G]
Throat – sore
Tongue – ulcers [G]
Vomiting
Vomiting – blood (hematemesis) [G]

Differentiation

Includes, but not limited to:
    Brown recluse spider bite
    Cat-scratch disease
    Cellulitis
    Congestive heart failure [19]
    Cowpox
    Cutaneous diphtheria
    Influenza
    Orf

Plague
Rickettsial infection
Staphylococcal disease
Tularemia
Upper respiratory infection

Complications
Include, but not limited to:
Atrial fibrillation [23]
Hemorrhagic meningitis
Hemorrhagic necrotizing mediastinitis [I] [7]
Hyperkalemia
Hypocalcemia
Hypoglycemia
Microangiopathic hemolytic anemia [21]
Respiratory failure [I]
Subarachnoid hemorrhage
Shock

Laboratory [32] ▲
Blood arterial pH – decreased (acidosis)
Blood arterial pO_2 – decreased (hypoxia)
Blood bacterial culture – positive
Blood bacterial stain – positive
Blood creatinine – increased
Blood immunoabsorbent assay – positive
Blood liver enzymes – increased
Blood sodium – decreased
Blood serum creatinine, total – increased
Blood WBC – left shift
Blood WBC total – increased (leukocytosis) [28]
CSF bacterial culture – positive
CSF bacterial stain – positive
CSF – blood
CSF RBC – increased
Pleural fluid, bacterial culture – positive
Pleural fluid, bacterial stain – positive
Pleural fluid – blood
Skin lesion, bacterial culture – positive
Skin lesion, bacterial stain – positive

Sputum bacterial culture – positive
Sputum bacterial stain – positive

ECG
Abnormalities – NS
Voltage, gen – decreased [33]

Imaging [I] [18, 25]
Heart, pericardium – fluid
Hilar adenopathy – bilateral
Lungs, hilar lymph nodes – enlarged
Lungs, parenchyma – consolidation
Lungs, parenchyma – infiltrates
Lungs, peribronchi – thickened
Lungs, pleura – fluid
Mediastinum – enlarged [10]

Other Tests
Skin lesion punch biopsy [C] [26]
Thoracentesis – hemorrhagic pleural effusion [I]

Treatment – Nonpharmacologic
Fluids and electrolytes
Ventilation

Treatment – Pharmacologic
Antibiotics [27]
      Chloramphenicol
      Doxycycline
      Erythromycin
      Fluroquinolones
      Penicillin

Treatment – Surgical/Invasive
NA in absence of complications

Precautions [32] ▲
Airborne
Protective clothing [5]
Site decontamination

Spore contact ▲
Standard

Primary Prevention

Vaccine: yes [4]
Postexposure prophylaxis
    Ciprofloxacin
    Doxycycline
Standard
Transmission barriers [32] ▲

Course

Untreated

Cutaneous – 20% fatal ☠
Gastrointestinal – 25–60% fatal ☠
Inhalational – 100% fatal ☠

Treated [9]

Cutaneous – mortality <10%
Gastrointestinal – unknown
Inhalational – 60% cured in post 9-11 cases, but much higher mortality in prior series of natural outbreaks

Notes

[1]   May resemble acute abdomen
[2]   Tender
[3]   Depressed, painless black eschar
[4]   2 doses AVA vaccine effective for aerosol exposure
[5]   Mask: US military m17 & m40 protect against 1-5 um particles
[6]   Large aerobic, gram-positive sporulating rod
[7]   Necropsy finding, virtually diagnostic of anthrax
[8]   Esp face, arms, hands
[9]   Variable depending on when therapy started
[10]   Due to hyperdense, enlarged mediastinal adenopathy and diffuse mediastinal edema
[11]   May resemble mosquito bite
[12]   Gelatinous, nonpitting
[13]   May be pronounced on face
[14]   Skin lesion may be small or absent
[15]   May be disproportionate to fever or symptoms

[16] Not typical, but reported with blood-tinged sputum in 2001 USA outbreak

[17] Based on 2001 USA outbreak, clinical presentation of intentional infection may vary from classical descriptions

[18] Noncontrast CT may be more useful than contrast CT to detect hyperdense adenopathy

[19] Initial treatment of case reported in 2001 USA outbreak

[20] "Anthrax" derived from greek *anthrakos* for "coal," in reference to black eschar typical of cutaneous form

[21] Reported in infant in 2001 USA outbreak

[22] May be minimal, as in some cases in 2001

[23] Uncommon, reported in 1 case of inhalational form in 2001

[24] Includes signs/symptoms of inhalational form in 2001

[25] Some form of abnormality present in 10/10 inhalational forms in 2001; pleural effusion most common (8/10)

[26] Obtain prior to antibiotic when possible

[27] Antibiotics that show in vitro effectiveness and may be considered if for any reason penicillin, fluroquinolones, or tetracyclines cannot be used, or for augmentation, include: chloramphenicol, clindamycin, extended-spectrum penicillins, macrolides, aminoglycosides, vancomycin, cefazolin, other first-generation cephalosporins

[28] May be normal

[29] Active infection occurs with toxin release from bacillary form

[30] Within envelopes delivered by mail

[31] Reported childhood cases rare

[32] BSL-3 standards ▲

[33] When pericardial effusion present

[34] Due to mesenteric adenopathy

http://www.argus1.com/?anthrax

Updates

_____
_____
_____
_____
_____
_____
_____
_____
_____

Avian Influenza

Weapon
No

Alternate Names
Bird flu

Etiology
Influenza virus A subtype H5N1

Intracelluar viral replication in upper and lower respiratory tract within 24 hours after infection; present in secretions for 3-5 days; edema and hyperemia of upper and lower respiratory cells, esp bronchial epithelial cells, with loss of cilia; extends to alveolar cells in pneumonia

Transmission
Source: Birds – wild and domestic
Entry: Inhalation
Human-to-Human: Rare [5] ▲

Predisposing/Comorbid Conditions
NA

Demographics [5]
Location: Influenza A H5N1 infections in Republic of Korea, Vietnam, Japan, Tapei China, Thailand, Cambodia, Hong Kong, Laos, Indonesia, People's Republic of China; other types reported in past in Virginia (H5N2 Shenandoah Valley, 2002; H7N7 Netherlands, 2003; H7N3, Canada, 2004)
Populations: All, esp persons exposed to poultry [4]
Calendar: Year-round

Systems

Gastrointestinal
Musculoskeletal
Optic
Oropharynx
Respiratory – lower
Respiratory – upper

Incubation

Up to 10 days

Signs/Symptoms [2]

Abdomen – pain
Appetite – reduced (anorexia)
Bowel movements – diarrhea
Chest, ant – pain, pleuritic
Chills
Cough – nonproductive
Cough – productive
Dizziness (lightheaded)
Eyes, conjunctivae – injected
Eyes, motion – painful
Eyes, tears (lacrimation) – excess
Eyes, vision – light sensitivity, increased (photophobia)
Face, parotid glands – enlarged
Fatigue
Head – pain (headache)
Joints – pain (arthralgia)
Lymph nodes, ant cervical – enlarged
Mentation – weakness (malaise)
Muscles – pain (myalgia)
Muscles – stiffness
Muscles – tender
Nausea
Nose, mucosa – inflamed
Nose – congested
Nose – drainage (rhinorrhea, coryza)
Temperature, body – elevated (fever)
Throat – dry
Throat – injected

Throat – sore
Voice – hoarse
Vomiting

Differentiation
Includes, but not limited to:
Numerous other viral and bacterial infectious diseases with malaise,
    headache, fever, myalgia, sore throat, early in course.

Complications [2]
Include, but not limited to:
Encephalopathy/encephalitis
Guillain-Barré syndrome
Myelitis
Myocarditis
Myositis
Pericarditis
Pneumonia – bacterial
Pneumonia – viral
Reye's syndrome
Rhabdomyolysis
Toxic shock syndrome

Laboratory [1] ▲
Blood lymphocytes – decreased (lymphopenia)

ECG
NA in absence of myocarditis, pericarditis, or other complications
    [2]

Imaging
NA in absence of pulmonary or other complications [2]

Other Tests
NA in absence of complications [2]

Treatment – Nonpharmacologic
Fluids and electrolytes

Treatment – Pharmacologic
Antivirals [3]
Symptomatic [6] ▲

Treatment – Surgical/Invasive
NA in absence of complications

Precautions
See [1] ▲

Primary Prevention
Avoidance/control of infected animals and secretions

Course
Variable
More severe in elderly and persons with preexisting conditions
Often fatal ☠ [5]

Notes
[1]   CDC: "Highly pathogenic avian influenza A (H5N1) is classified as a select agent and must be worked with under BSL 3+ laboratory conditions. This includes controlled access double door entry with change room and shower, use of respirators, decontamination of all wastes, and showering out of all personnel. Laboratories working on these viruses must be certified by the US Department of Agriculture. The same BSL 3+ laboratory guidelines are recommended for conducting virus isolation for SARS-CoV. CDC does not recommend that virus isolation studies on respiratory specimens from patients who meet the above criteria be conducted unless stringent BSL 3+ conditions can be met. Therefore, respiratory virus cultures should not be performed in most clinical laboratories and such cultures should not be ordered for patients suspected of having H5N1 infection." ▲

[2]   Mainly based on data derived from common influenza, but case reports to date indicate that respiratory involvement may be more prominent in Avian influenza

[3]   Uncertain, variable efficacy; consult current guidelines

[4]   Contact with wild birds, ducks, chickens, turkeys, or (unproven) infected humans

[5]   To publication date ▲

[6]   Avoid aspirin and aspirin-containing products for febrile infections in children <19 yrs due to association with Reye's syndrome

http://www.argus1.com/?avian

Updates

_____

_____

_____

_____

_____

_____

_____

_____

_____

_____

_____

_____

_____

_____

_____

_____

_____

_____

_____

Bolivian Hemorrhagic Fever

Weapon
CDC Bioterrorism Category: A

Alternate Names
Black typhus
Machupo virus
South American hemorrhagic fever

Etiology
Machupo virus [5]

Transmission
Source:	Rodents, esp vesper mouse
Entry:	Inhalation
	Contact
Human-to-Human:	Yes (uncommon)

Predisposing/Comorbid Conditions
NA

Demographics
Location:	Bolivia
Populations:	All
Calendar:	Year-round, peak April-July

Systems
Circulatory
Coagulation
Nervous

Incubation
7-16 days

Signs/Symptoms [4]

Abdomen – pain
Appetite – reduced (anorexia)
Arterial press – low
Back – pain [3]
Bowel movements, stool – blood or black (hematochezia) (melena)
Bowel movements – constipation
Dizziness (lightheaded)
Eyes, retroorbital – pain
Eyes, vision – light sensitivity, increased (photophobia)
Face – flushed
Head – pain (headache)
Heart rate – slow (bradycardia)
Mentation – weakness (malaise)
Mouth, mucosa – petechiae
Muscles – pain (myalgia)
Muscles – tremors, intention
Nausea
Nose – blood (epistaxis) [1]
Skin, upper body – flushed, erythematous
Skin – rash, petechiae [2]
Temperature, body – elevated (fever)
Tendon reflexes, gen – reduced or absent
Throat – red, injected
Urine – blood (hematuria)
Vomiting
Vomiting – blood (hematemesis) [1]

Differentiation

Includes, but not limited to:
Lassa fever
Lymphocytic choriomeningitis
Other causes of encephalitis
Other viral hemorrhagic fevers

Complications

Shock

Laboratory [6] ▲
Blood culture – positive
Blood IgM enzyme assay – positive
Blood platelets – decreased (thrombocytopenia)
Blood WBC – decreased (leukopenia)
Urine – casts, cellular
Urine protein – present (proteinuria)
Urine RBC – present (hematuria, microhematuria)

ECG
NA in absence of complications

Imaging
NA in absence of complications

Other Tests
NA in absence of complications

Treatment – Nonpharmacologic
Fluids and electrolytes

Treatment – Pharmacologic
Immune plasma
Ribavirin

Treatment – Surgical/Invasive
NA

Precautions
Standard

Primary Prevention
Vaccine: no
Rodent control

Course
Mortality 15-30% ☠

Notes

[1] Early in course
[2] Esp upper trunk
[3] May be severe
[4] Other symptoms of encephalitis may also occur
[5] Member of Tacaribe complex of arenaviruses
[6] BSL-4 procedures ▲

http://www.argus1.com/?bolivian

Updates

_____
_____
_____
_____
_____
_____
_____
_____
_____
_____
_____
_____
_____
_____
_____
_____
_____
_____
_____
_____

Botulism

Weapon
CDC Bioterrorism Category: A

Alternate Names
Foodborne botulism (F)
Infant botulism
Intestinal botulism (I)
Wound botulism (W)

Etiology
Toxin of *clostridium botulinum* [9]

Disseminates from initial body site via blood and lymphatics to nerve terminals, blocking release of acetylcholine at neuromuscular junctions, ganglionic nerve endings, and postganglionic parasympathetic and sympathetic nerve endings

Transmission

Sources [21]:	(I) Toxins produced in large intestine following ingestion of spore-contaminated food or soil
	(F) Ingestion of food contaminated with preformed toxin [20]
	(W) Toxins formed in wounds under anaerobic conditions
Entry:	Ingestion
	Contact
Human-to-Human:	No

Predisposing/Comorbid Conditions [18]
Abscess [26]
Altered GI flora
Illicit IV and subcutaneous drug use

Post-surgery
Wounds

Demographics
Populations: All
Locations: Global
Calendar: Year-round

Systems [17]
Gastrointestinal
Nervous
Optic

Incubation
Hours

Signs/Symptoms [11, 23, 25]
Abdomen – distention
Abdomen – pain [1, 2]
Appearance, gen – "floppy"
Bladder, urinary – distention
Bowel movements – constipation [2, 24] ▲
Bowel movements – diarrhea [13]
Bowel sounds – decreased/absent (ileus, adynamic)
Breathing, rest – difficult (rest dyspnea)
Breathing – irregular
Cranial nerve III – palsy
Cranial nerve IV – palsy
Cranial nerve VI – palsy
Dizziness (lightheadedness)
Extremities – pain, shooting (paresthesias)
Eyes, gaze – paralysis
Eyes, lids – drooping (ptosis) [6]
Eyes, motion – jerky (nystagmus) [6]
Eyes, motion – wandering (strabismus) [6]
Eyes, pupil reaction – sluggish [6]
Eyes, pupils – dilation (mydriasis) [6]
Eyes, vision – blurred
Eyes, vision – double (diplopia)
Face, muscles bilat – weak/paralyzed [6]

Mentation – conscious
Mentation – fatigue
Gait – ataxic
Head – pain (headache)
Heart rate – slow (bradycardia) [12]
Mood – anxious
Mood – lethargic
Mouth – dry (xerostomia)
Muscles, tone – decreased (hypotonia) [6]
Muscles – paralysis [3, 6]
Muscles – weak [6]
Nausea
Neck, muscle control – decreased/absent
Speech, voice – changed (dysphonia)
Speech – disturbed (dysphasia)
Speech – inarticulate (dysarthria)
Swallowing – difficult (dysphagia)
Temperature, body – normal [8]
Tendon reflexes – decreased/absent [6]
Throat, gag reflex – absent
Throat – injected
Throat – sore
Tongue – enlarged (macroglossia)
Tongue – weakness
Vomiting

Differentiation [22] ▲

Includes, but not limited to:
Acute abdomen
Anticholinergic poisoning
Carbon monoxide poisoning
Chemical/drug poisoning [14]
Diphtheria
Food poisoning [15]
Guillain-Barré syndrome [5] ▲
Lambert-Eaton myasthenic-myotonic syndrome
Myasthenia gravis
Organophosphate poisoning
Poliomyelitis
Stroke

Tetanus
Tick paralysis

Complications
Include, but not limited to:
Pneumonia
Respiratory failure

Laboratory [16]
Blood toxin – positive [7]
Gastric aspirate toxin – positive [F] [7]
Stool toxin – positive [7]
Wound culture – positive [W]
Wound toxin – positive [W] [7]

ECG
Rate – slow (sinus bradycardia) [12]

Imaging
NA in absence of complications

Other Tests
Continuous cardiac and respiratory monitoring with suspected
diagnosis
EMG – characteristic low amplitude pattern in affected muscles
Rapid detection environmental tests

Treatment – Nonpharmacologic
Fluids and electrolytes
Gastric and colonic lavage [F]
Respiratory support

Treatment – Pharmacologic [27]
Antitoxin [28]
Guanidine

Treatment – Surgical/Invasive
NA in absence of complications

Precautions
Standard

Primary Prevention
Vaccine: yes
Do not feed honey to infants under 1 year ▲
Proper food preparation and preservation

Course
Variable
Treated mortality <5%
Untreated often fatal ☠

Notes
[1]   Cramping
[2]   May be severe
[3]   Descending, flaccid
[4]   Reduced amplitude evoked potentials; increased amplitude with rapid repetitive nerve stimulation
[5]   Most common misdiagnosis ▲
[6]   Neurologic abnormalities symmetrical
[7]   Obtain before giving antitoxin
[8]   Differentiation from many other infections
[9]   Spore-forming anaerobe with 7 toxins (A-G)
[10]   Esp honey and home-canned foods
[11]   Onset varies according to type
[12]   Rate may be normal
[13]   Occurs early in course
[14]   Carbon monoxide, barium carbonate, methyl chloride, methyl alcohol, organic phosphate compounds, atropine, aminoglycosides, neomycin, streptomycin, kanamycin, gentamicin
[15]   Many other forms, i.e., salmonellosis, *clostridium perfringens*, staphylotoxin, etc
[16]   Most tests to exclude other etiologies
[17]   Toxin absorbed through skin wound or intestinal or lung mucosa and carried via blood to neuromuscular junctions, blocking acetylcholine release beginning in bulbar musculature
[18]   Intestinal form usually occurs in infants or adults with prior GI disease

[19]   Formerly termed "infant botulism"

[20]   Home-canned foods, honey, puffer fish, paralytic shellfish, mushrooms

[21]   Global presence of spores in soil, animals, fish, marine sediment, agricultural products

[22]   Botulism may be confused with many other entities ▲

[23]   Key features: afebrile; symmetrical neurological deficits; bradycardia; conscious; no sensory loss

[24]   May be initial finding, lasting for weeks before other symptoms, in infants ▲

[25]   Also with weak cry, poor/absent feeding, etc, in infants

[26]   I.e., sinus, tooth

[27]   Do not give aminogycoside antibiotics, which increase neuromuscular blockade ▲

[28]   Early administration important for survival ▲

http://www.argus1.com/?botulism

Updates

_____
_____
_____
_____
_____
_____
_____
_____
_____
_____
_____
_____
_____
_____
_____
_____
_____
_____
_____
_____
_____

Brucellosis

Weapon
CDC Bioterrorism Category: B

Alternate Names
Cyprus fever
Gibraltar fever
Malta fever
Mediterranean fever
Rock fever
Undulant fever

Etiology
B mellitensis (most cases)
B abortus
B suis
B canis

Phagocytyzed, multiply and spread in lymphatics within WBCs and macrophages to regional lymph nodes, then into bloodstream in systemic acute infection; chronic reaction to form granulomas, esp in liver, spleen and other reticuloendothelial tissue, with fibrosis and calcification after healing.

Transmission
Sources:	Cattle, goats, dogs, pigs, sheep, deer, horses, camels, moose, rabbits, chickens, infected human milk
Entry:	Ingestion [7]
	Contact
	Inhalation
	Organ transplantation
Human-to-Human:	Rare except breast feeding

Predisposing/Comorbid Conditions
Skin abrasion

Demographic

Populations:	All, esp occupations in contact with infected animals, such as butchers and veterinarians
Location:	Global
Calendar:	Year-round

Systems

Gastrointestinal
Liver/biliary tract/pancreas
Lymphatic
Musculoskeletal
Nervous

Incubation

5-60 days

Signs/Symptoms [2]

Abdomen – pain
Appetite – reduced (anorexia)
Back, cervical – pain
Back, lumbar – pain
Bowel movements – constipation [4]
Bowel movements – diarrhea [3]
Chills
Head – pain (headache)
Joints – pain (arthralgia)
Liver – enlarged (hepatomegaly)
Lymph nodes – enlarged
Mentation – fatigue
Mentation – feeling of weakness (malaise)
Mood – depressed
Mood – labile
Mood – restless/irritable
Muscles – pain (myalgia)
Sleep – disturbed (insomnia)
Spleen – enlarged (splenomegaly)
Sweating – increased (hyperhidrosis)
Temperature, body – elevated (fever) [8]
Weight – loss

Differentiation
Includes, but not limited to:
    Chronic fatigue syndrome [5]
    Influenza
    Other causes of systemic infection

Complications [9]
Include, but not limited to:
    Anemia
    Arthritis
    Bleeding
    Chronic brucellosis
    Endocarditis [1]
    Epididymoorchitis
    Episcleritis
    Genitourinary infection
    Hepatitis
    Leukopenia
    Meningoencephalitis
    Myelitis
    Neuropathy
    Osteomyelitis
    Papilledema
    Prostate infection
    Pulmonary infection
    Radiculitis
    Splenic abscess
    Thrombocytopenia
    Uveitis

Laboratory [6] ▲
    Blood culture – positive
    Blood Hgb, Hct – decreased (anemia)
    Blood IgG antibodies – increased
    Blood liver enzymes – increased
    Blood platelets – decreased (thrombocytopenia)
    Blood WBC – decreased (leukopenia)
    Bone marrow culture – positive
    CSF culture – positive

Tissue biopsy culture – positive
Urine culture – positive

ECG
NA in absence of complications

Imaging
NA in absence of complications

Other Tests
NA in absence of complications

Treatment – Nonpharmacologic
NS

Treatment – Pharmacologic
Combined doxycycline and rifampin, streptomycin, or gentamycin

Treatment – Surgical/Invasive
Abscess drainage
NA except for complication, esp abscess drainage, splenectomy

Precautions
Careful handling of all specimens [6] ▲

Primary Prevention
Vaccine: no
Animal immunization
Pasteurization

Course
Full recovery usual in 2-3 weeks
Rarely fatal [1]

Notes
[1]   Endocarditis is most common cause of death ☠
[2]   Typically there may be many symptoms, but few physical signs
[3]   At onset only, with constipation predominant thereafter

[4]   May be severe
[5]   Chronic form
[6]   BSL-3 laboratory handling requires extreme care ▲
[7]   Esp unpasteurized milk and cheese
[8]   May occur in waves – "undulent"
[9]   May become focal and persistent

http://www.argus1.com/?bruce

Updates

_____
_____
_____
_____
_____
_____
_____
_____
_____
_____
_____
_____
_____
_____
_____
_____
_____
_____
_____
_____

Campylobacteriosis

Weapon
No

Alternate Names
Campylobacter enteritis

Etiology
Campylobacter jejuni [1]

Transmission
Source: Contaminated food (esp poultry), water, animals (esp cats, puppies)
Entry: Ingestion
Human-to-Human: Rare

Predisposing/Comorbid Conditions
More severe in immune compromise

Demographic
Location: Global
Populations: All, esp infants and young adults
              Males>females
Calendar: Summer>winter

Systems
Gastrointestinal

Incubation
2-5 days

Signs/Symptoms
Abdomen – cramps

Abdomen – pain [3]
Abdomen – tenderness
Bowel movements, stool – blood or black (hematochezia) (melena)
Bowel movements, stool – mucoid
Bowel movements – diarrhea
Head – pain (headache) [2]
Muscles – pain (myalgia) [2]
Nausea
Temperature, body – elevated (fever) [2]
Vomiting

Differentiation
Includes, but not limited to:
Appendicitis
Gastroenteritis – other causes
Pancreatitis

Complications
Include, but not limited to:
Arthritis [5]
Dehydration
Endocarditis [4] [5]
Guillain-Barré syndrome [5]
Meningitis [5]
Sepsis with secondary infection of gallbladder, pancreas, bone [5]
Toxic megacolon

Laboratory
Stool blood – positive
Stool culture – positive
Stool direct identification of bacteria
Stool mucus – increased
Stool WBC – increased

ECG
NS in absence of complications

Imaging
NS in absence of complications

Other Tests
NS in absence of complications

Treatment – Nonpharmacologic
Fluids and electrolytes

Treatment – Pharmacologic [6]
Antibiotics
>Aminoglycoside
>Erythromycin
>Fluroquinolone
>Tetracycline

Treatment – Surgical/Invasive
NA in absence of complications

Precautions
Handwashing, other barrier techniques ▲

Primary Prevention
Avoid contaminated water
Handwashing after handling raw poultry
Milk pasteurization
Prevention of kitchen cross-contamination
Thorough cooking of poultry products

Course
Recovery usual, with some cases of relapse reported

Notes
[1]   Most common bacterial cause of diarrhea in USA
[2]   Prodromal period of 1-2 days preceding diarrhea
[3]   May be severe, more prominent than diarrhea, resembling appendicitis, pancreatitis
[4]   ESP *c fetus*
[5]   ESP immune compromise, i.e., AIDS, cancer
[6]   For severe symptoms, early in course

http://www.argus1.com/?campy

Updates

_____

_____

_____

_____

_____

_____

_____

_____

_____

_____

_____

_____

_____

_____

_____

_____

_____

_____

_____

_____

_____

_____

_____

Chickenpox

Weapon
No

Alternate Names
Varicella
VZV

Etiology
Varicella-zoster virus

Viral replication in mucosal cells of upper respiratory tract followed by viremia and skin infection

Transmission [11]

Source:	Infected human vesicular fluid, upper respiratory tract secretions
Entry:	Inhalation
	Maternal – fetal
Human-to-Human:	Yes

Predisposing/Comorbid Conditions
More severe in immune compromise (i.e., leukemia, lymphoma, HIV, corticosteroids treatment)

Demographic

Location:	Global
Populations:	All [10]
Calendar:	Temperate climate peak in late winter – early spring

Systems [8]
Oropharynx

Respiratory – upper
Skin

Incubation

10-21 days

Signs/Symptoms

Anorectum – vesicles
Appetite – reduced (anorexia)
Chest – cough, acute, NS [6]
Eyes, conjunctivae – vesicles
Head – pain (headache)
Lymph nodes, post cervical – enlarged [1]
Lymph nodes, suboccipital – enlarged [1]
Mouth, mucosa – vesicles
Muscles – pain (myalgia)
Nose – drainage (rhinorrhea, coryza)
Skin – itching (pruritus)
Skin – rash, crusting [3]
Skin – rash, macular/papular [2, 3]
Skin – rash, pustular [3]
Skin – rash, vesicular [3, 4]
Swallowing – pain (odynophagia) [5]
Temperature, body – elevated (fever) [12]
Throat – sore
Vagina – vesicles
Voice – hoarse [6]

Differentiation

Includes, but not limited to:
Drug rash
Enterovirus infection
Erythropoietic porphyria
Generalized herpes in immune compromise
Guttate psoriasis
Impetigo
Insect bites
Rickettsialpox
Secondary syphilis
Smallpox

Complications
Include, but not limited to:
    Arthritis – septic
    Benign cerebellar ataxis
    Dehydration
    Disseminated intravascular coagulation
    Encephalitis
    Fetal malformations
    Guillain-Barré syndrome
    Intracranial vasculitis
    Myocarditis
    Nephritis
    Optic neuritis
    Osteomyelitis
    Pneumonia – interstitial
    Pyoderma
    Reye's syndrome [7]
    Secondary bacterial skin infection
    Thrombocytopenia
    Transverse myelitis
    Vasculitis

Laboratory
Blood serology – positive

ECG
NA in absence of complications

Imaging [9]
NA in absence of complications

Other Tests
Skin culture for secondary infection

Treatment – Nonpharmacologic
Skin hygiene
Trim nails

Treatment – Pharmacologic [13]
Acetaminophen

Acyclovir
Antipruritics

Treatment – Surgical/Invasive
NA in absence of complications

Precautions
Isolation until encrustation of skin lesions ▲
Standard

Primary Prevention
Vaccine: yes
Varicella-zoster immune globulin (VZIG)

Course
Full recovery usual
More severe in adults and immune compromise
Self-limited

Notes
[1]   Secondary to scalp lesions
[2]   Accompanied by evanescent flush
[3]   Begins on head, quickly spreading to trunk and arms; palms and soles of feet rare; occurs in crops
[4]   On red areola; more prominent in adults
[5]   Due to throat vesicles
[6]   Due to laryngotracheitis
[7]   Less common with aspirin avoidance
[8]   Initial viral replication in mucosal cells of upper respiratory tract, followed by viremia and skin infection; reactivation as herpes zoster in later years
[9]   Chest x-ray when pneumonia suspected: diffuse nodular infiltrates, hilar adenopathy, pleural effusion
[10] In temperate climates, usually children; in tropics, usually adults
[11] Contagious 1-2 days before symptom onset until rash is fully encrusted
[12] Concurrent with rash onset
[13] Avoid aspirin-related products, which cause Reye's syndrome ▲

Updates

_____

_____

_____

_____

_____

_____

_____

_____

_____

_____

_____

_____

_____

_____

_____

_____

_____

_____

_____

_____

_____

Cholera

Weapon
CDC Bioterrorism Category: B

Alternate Names
NA

Etiology
V. cholerae (gram-neg bacteria)

Toxin binds to GI epithelial cells causing excessive fluid secretion and sodium and water malabsorption

Transmission
Source: Infected water, undercooked fish or vegetables washed in contaminated water

Entry: Ingestion

Human-to-Human: Yes (fecal-oral)

Predisposing/Comorbid Conditions
Blood group type O
H pylori infection

Demographics
Location: Global

Populations: Impoverished and children under age 5 years most often affected where disease is common; disaster victims

Calendar: Year-round, peak in hot seasons

Systems
Gastrointestinal

Incubation
1-7 days

Signs/Symptoms [3, 4]

Abdomen – cramps
Abdomen – distension [6]
Arterial pressure – decreased
Arterial pulse, amplitude – decreased/absent
Bowel movements – diarrhea [1]
Bowel sounds – decreased/absent (ileus, adynamic) [6]
Bowel sounds – increased
Breathing – rapid, deep (tachypnea)
Consciousness – loss, prolonged (coma)
Eyes – dry
Eyes – sunken
Heart, rate – rapid (tachycardia)
Heart sounds, intensity – decreased
Mentation – anxious
Mentation – apathy
Mentation – fatigue
Mentation – sleepy (somnolence)
Mood – depressed
Mood – lethargic
Mouth – dry (xerostomia)
Muscles – cramps
Nausea
Seizures
Skin turgor – decreased
Thirst – excessive
Urine volume – decreased (oliguria)
Voice – hoarse
Vomiting

Differentiation

Includes, but not limited to:

All other causes of gastroenteritis

Complications

Include, but not limited to:

Hypoglycemia
Hypovolemic shock
Metabolic acidosis
Noncardiac pulmonary edema

Pneumonia
Renal failure
Sepsis
Spontaneous abortion

Laboratory

Blood arterial pH – decreased (acidosis)
Blood concentration – increased
Blood culture – positive
Blood glucose – decreased [7]
Blood glucose – increased
Blood potassium – decreased (hypokalemia) [2]
Stool bacterial stain – positive
Stool culture – positive
WBC – increased (leukocytosis)

ECG

NS changes

Imaging

NA in absence of complications

Other Tests

NA in absence of complications

Treatment – Nonpharmacologic

Fluids and electrolytes

Treatment – Pharmacologic [5]

Antibiotics
        Doxycycline
        Tetracycline

Treatment – Surgical/Invasive

NA in absence of complications

Precautions

Enteric
Standard

Primary Prevention

Vaccine: yes
Hygiene
Proper food preparation
Water purification

Course

Variable
Mortality up to 60% ☠

Notes

[1]   Painless, watery, abrupt
[2]   Not apparent until acidosis corrected
[3]   Most infected persons are asymptomatic
[4]   Many due to dehydration
[5]   Resistance is common and role of antibiotics uncertain
[6]   Cholera sicca
[7]   Poorer prognosis

http://www.argus1.com/?cholera

Updates

_____
_____
_____
_____
_____
_____
_____
_____
_____
_____
_____
_____
_____
_____
_____
_____
_____
_____

Clostridium Perfringens Gastroenteritis

Weapon
No [2]

Alternate Names
Food poisoning

Etiology
Clostridium perfringens

Transmission
Source: Contaminated food and water
Entry: Ingestion
Human-to-Human: No

Predisposing/Comorbid Conditions
NA

Demographics
Location: Global
Populations: All
Calendar: Year-round

Systems
Gastrointestinal

Incubation
6-24 hours

Signs/Symptoms
Abdomen – pain
Appetite – decreased (anorexia)

Bowel movements – diarrhea
Nausea [1]

Differentiation
Includes, but not limited to:
Other causes of gastroenteritis and food poisoning

Complications
Include but not limited to:
Dehydration
Necrotizing enteritis
Septicemia

ECG
NA in absence of complications

Laboratory
NA in absence of complications

Imaging
NA in absence of complications

Other Tests
NA in absence of complications

Treatment – Nonpharmacologic
Fluids and electrolytes

Treatment – Pharmacologic
NS

Treatment – Surgical/Invasive
NA in absence of complications

Precautions
Standard

Primary Prevention
Food handling and preparation

Course
Self-limited

Notes
[1]   Vomiting usually not present
[2]   Epsilon toxin of *clostridium perfringens*, however, has been identified as a possible bioweapon

http://www.argus1.com/?closgas

Updates

_____

_____

_____

_____

_____

_____

_____

_____

_____

_____

_____

_____

_____

_____

_____

_____

_____

_____

_____

_____

_____

Crimean – Congo Hemorrhagic Fever

Weapon
CDC Bioterrorism Category: A

Alternate Names
Central Asian hemorrhagic fever

Etiology
Bunyaviridae virus

Generalized vascular damage and endothelial lesions, followed by disseminated intravascular coagulation and formation of microthrombi with subsequent tissue infarction

Transmission
Source:	Ticks, large and small animals including birds and livestock; human blood/secretions; infected animals
Entry:	Insect bite
	Ingestion
Human-to-Human:	Yes

Predisposing/Comorbid Conditions
NA

Demographics
Location:	Rural Asia, Eastern Europe, Africa
Populations:	Farmers, veterinarians, laboratory personnel
Calendar:	Seasonal variations correlate with tick activity

Systems
Cardiovascular
Coagulation

Gastrointestinal
Liver/biliary tract/pancreas
Nervous
Oropharynx
Reticuloendothelial

Incubation
2-7 days

Signs/Symptoms [1]
Abdomen, epigastrium – pain
Abdomen, RUQ – pain
Abdomen – pain
Appetite – decreased (anorexia)
Back – pain
Bowel movements – diarrhea
Bowel movements – blood or black (melena)
Breath sounds – crackling (rales) [2]
Chills
Dizziness (lightheaded)
Eyes, conjunctivae – injected
Eyes, vision – light sensitivity, increased (photophobia)
Eyes – pain
Face – flushed
Head – pain (headache)
Heart rate – rapid (tachycardia)
Heart rate – slow (bradycardia)
Liver – enlarged (hepatomegaly)
Lymph nodes – enlarged
Mentation – confusion
Mentation – sleepiness (somnolence)
Mentation – weakness (malaise)
Mood – depressed
Mood – labile
Mood – lethargic
Mood – restless/irritable
Mouth, gingiva – bleeding
Mouth, mucosa – petechiae
Mouth, palate – petechiae
Muscles – pain (myalgia)

Nausea
Neck, post – pain
Neck, post – stiff (meningismus)
Nose – bleeding (epistaxis)
Skin – ecchymoses
Skin – rash, petechiae
Sputum – blood (hemoptysis)
Temperature, body – elevated (fever)
Throat – injected
Throat – petechiae
Throat – sore
Urine – blood (hematuria)
Vomiting
Vomiting – blood (hematemesis)

Differentiation
Includes, but not limited to:
    Clotting disorders
    Encephalitis
    Other viral hemorrhagic fevers

Complications
Include, but not limited to:
    Anemia
    Circulatory collapse
    Disseminated intravascular coagulation
    Hepatic failure
    Massive hemorrhage
    Renal failure

Laboratory [3] ▲
    Blood fibrinogen – decreased
    Blood IgG antibodies – positive
    Blood IgM antibodies – positive
    Blood liver enzymes – increased
    Blood platelets – decreased (thrombocytopenia)
    Blood PTT – increased
    Blood WBC – decreased (leukopenia)

ECG
    Rate – increased (sinus tachycardia)

Imaging
NA in absence of complications

Other Tests
NA in absence of complications

Treatment – Nonpharmacologic
Blood replacement
Fluids and electrolytes

Treatment – Pharmacologic
Ribavirin

Treatment – Surgical/Invasive
NA in absence of complications

Precautions
Handling specimens [3] ▲
Standard

Primary Prevention
Vaccine: no
Tick control/avoidance

Course
Untreated
Mortality 30% ☠

Notes
[1]   Course typically consists of initial phase with abrupt onset of signs and symptoms lasting 3-5 days, followed by overtly hemorrhagic phase
[2]   Pulmonary edema
[3]   BSL-4 procedures ▲

http://www.argus1.com/?crimean

Updates

_____
_____
_____
_____
_____
_____
_____
_____
_____
_____
_____
_____
_____
_____
_____
_____
_____
_____
_____
_____
_____

Cryptosporidiosis

Weapon
CDC Bioterrorism Category: B

Alternate Names
Crypto

Etiology
Cryptosporidium parvum

Oocytes enter brush border of intestinal epithelium, develop into merozoites and multiply, impairing absorption of glucose, electrolytes, water, and fats, and vitamin B12 in severe cases

Transmission
Source:	Water and food contaminated by feces from humans and domestic animals
Entry:	Ingestion
Human-to-Human:	Yes

Predisposing/Comorbid Conditions
Immune compromise

Demographics
Location:	Global
Populations:	All
Calendar:	Year-round

Systems
Gastrointestinal
Respiratory [10]

Incubation
2-14 days [9]

Signs/Symptoms [1, 8]

Abdomen – cramps
Abdomen – flatulence
Abdomen – pain
Abdomen – pain, after meals
Appetite – decreased (anorexia)
Bowel movements – diarrhea [2]
Breathing – difficult, rest (dyspnea) [10]
Muscles – pain (myalgia)
Nausea
Temperature, body – elevated (fever) [3]
Vomiting
Weight – loss

Differentiation

Includes, but not limited to:
All other forms of gastroenteritis

Complications

Include, but not limited to:
Cholangitis [4]
Cholecystitis [4]
Growth retardation
Malnutrition [11]
Pancreatitis [4]

Laboratory [6] ▲

Blood, antibodies – present
Blood concentration – increased (hemoconcentration)
Blood potassium – decreased
Stool oocytes – positive

ECG

NS abnormalities [5]

Imaging

Gallbladder – dilated [7]
Lungs – infiltrates [10]

Other Tests

Small bowel biopsy – oocytes in epithelium

Treatment – Nonpharmacologic
Fluids and electrolytes
Lactose-free diet

Treatment – Pharmacologic
Antimotility agents

Treatment – Surgical/Invasive
NA in absense of complications

Precautions
Handling of specimens [6] ▲
Standard

Primary Prevention
Vaccine: no
Contaminated water treatment/avoidance
Hygiene

Course
Clinical course lasts up to 14 days
Longer and sometimes fatal in immunocompromised patients ☠

Notes
[1]   Onset may be severe in some cases, esp in immune compromise
[2]   May be profuse, very watery; sometimes mucoid
[3]   Often afebrile
[4]   Esp in immune compromise
[5]   Due to electrolyte abnormalities
[6]   High incidence of transmission to health care workers when protective measures not taken ▲
[7]   Gallbladder imaging indicated if cholecystitis suspected
[8]   Carriers are often asymptomatic
[9]   Highly variable
[10]   Children, AIDS
[11]   Esp in developing countries

http://www.argus1.com/?crypto

Updates

Dengue

Weapon
No

Alternate Names
Breakbone fever
Dandy fever
Dengue fever
Dengue hemorrhagic fever [H]
Dengue shock syndrome [S]
Philippine hemorrhagic fever [H]
Southwest hemorrhagic fever [H]
Thai hemorrhagic fever [H]

Etiology
Dengue virus (a *Flavaridiae* virus)

Virus replicates in target organs such as local lymph nodes and liver, then released as a viremia, infecting WBC and lymphatic system and increasing vascular permeability causing massive fluid leakage

Transmission
Source: Mosquitoes, mainly *a aegypti*
Entry: Insect bite
Human-to-Human: No

Predisposing/Comorbid Conditions
NA

Demographic
Location: Global, esp tropics
Populations: All
Calendar: Year-round

Systems

Coagulation
Liver/biliary tract/pancreas
Musculoskeletal
Nervous
Optic
Oropharynx
Skin

Incubation

4-7 days

Signs/Symptoms

Abdomen – pain
Appetite – decreased (anorexia)
Arterial press – low
Arterial pulse press – narrow
Back, lumbar – pain
Bones – pain
Bowel movements, stool – blood or black (melena)
Chills
Cough – NS, acute
Eyes, conjunctivae – injected
Eyes, light sensitivity – increased (photophobia)
Eyes, retroorbital – pain
Eyes – tender
Face – flushed
Fatigue
Head, frontal – pain
Head – pain (headache) [1]
Heart rate – slow relative to fever (relative bradycardia)
Joints – pain (arthralgia)
Liver – enlarged (hepatomegaly)
Liver – tender
Lymph nodes, gen – enlarged
Menses, flow – increased (menorrhagia)
Mentation – confusion
Mood – depressed [2]
Mood – lethargic
Mood – restless, irritable

Mouth, gingiva – bleeding
Mouth, mucosa – ulcers
Mouth, soft palate – vesicles [3]
Muscles – pain (myalgia)
Muscles – paralysis
Muscles – weak [2]
Nausea
Neck, post – stiff (meningismus)
Nose – blood (epistaxis)
Nose – drainage (rhinorrhea)
Seizures
Sense of taste – altered
Sense of taste – bitter
Skin – rash, macular [4]
Skin – rash, petechiae
Skin – rash, purpura
Skin – rash, desquamating
Skin – red (erythema)
Skin – sensation increased (hyperesthesia)
Sleep – disturbed (insomnia)
Sputum – blood (hemoptysis)
Stools – black (melena)
Temperature, body – elevated (fever) [5]
Throat – sore
Urine – blood (hematuria)
Vomiting
Vomiting – blood (hematemesis)
Weight – loss

Differentiation
Includes, but not limited to:
Hepatitis
Influenza
Leptospirosis
Malaria
Other viral hemorrhagic fevers
Scrub typhus

Complications
Include, but not limited to:
Circulatory collapse [6]

Encephalitis
Gastric bleeding [7]
Hepatitis
Myocarditis
Neuropathy
Rhabdomyolysis

Laboratory
Blood concentration – increased
Blood liver enzymes – increased
Blood platelets – decreased (thrombocytopenia)
Blood serology – positive
Blood WBC – decreased (leukopenia)

Imaging
Abdomen – ascites
Lungs, pleura – fluid (pleural effusion)

Other Tests
Cell culture
Fluorescent antibody test
Tournequet test – positive

Treatment – Nonpharmacologic
Fluids and electrolytes
Fresh plasma
Oxygen
Plasma expanders

Treatment – Pharmacologic
Avoid aspirin ▲
NS

Treatment – Surgical/Invasive
NA in absence of complications

Precautions
Standard

Primary Prevention
Vaccine: in development
Vector control

Course
Variable

Notes
[1]   Aggravated by motion; typically frontal
[2]   Convalescent phase; may last for weeks
[3]   Microvesicles on post third
[4]   Esp chest, inner arms; spares palms and soles
[5]   Biphasic: initial fever abates in 3 days, with 2-3 day remission, then return of fever
[6]   Dengue hemorrhagic fever; children age 5 years and under
[7]   Esp with prior peptic ulcer disease

http://www..argus1.com/?dengue

Updates

_____
_____
_____
_____
_____
_____
_____
_____
_____
_____
_____
_____
_____
_____
_____
_____
_____
_____
_____
_____

E Coli 0l57:h7

Weapon
CDC Bioterrorism Category: B

Alternate Names
EHEC Shiga-producing *E coli*
STEC
Verotoxin-producing *E coli*
VTEC

Etiology
Toxins from (*E coli*) serotype 0157:h7 [7]

Bacteria adhere to intestinal epithelial cells with destruction of microvilli

Transmission
Source: Cattle, deer, human-contaminated water and food [2]
Entry: Ingestion
Human-to-Human: Yes (fecal-oral)

Predisposing/Comorbid Conditions
NA

Demographic
Location: Global
Populations: All, esp children under age 5 years and elderly
Calendar: Year-round

Systems
Gastrointestinal
Renal/Genitourinary

Incubation
2-8 days

Signs/Symptoms

Abdomen – pain
Bowel movements – blood or black (hematochezia) (melena)
Bowel movements – diarrhea [1]
Nausea
Vomiting

Differentiation

Includes, but not limited to:
Other causes of diarrhea [3]

Complications

Include, but not limited to:
Hemolytic uremic syndrome [4]
Thrombotic thrombocytopenic purpura

Laboratory

Stool blood – positive
Stool culture – positive [5]

ECG

NA in absence of complications

Imaging

NA in absence of complications

Other Tests

NA in absence of complications

Treatment – Nonpharmacologic

Fluids and electrolytes

Treatment – Pharmacologic

Avoid antidiarrheal agents ▲
NS

Treatment – Surgical/Invasive

NA

Precautions

Standard, esp enteric

Primary Prevention
Vaccine: cattle only
Avoid contaminated water
Hygiene
Proper food preparation
Water treatment

Course
Usual: recovery in 5-10 days

Notes
[1] Explosive, initially watery, becoming grossly bloody after a few days
[2] Contaminated water and inadequately cooked beef (esp ground beef), raw milk, fruit and vegetables
[3] Fever often present in other causes as differentiating point
[4] Occurs in 2-7% and is a major cause of renal failure in USA
[5] Specific request for this organism necessary

http://www.argus1.com/?ecoli015

Updates

_____
_____
_____
_____
_____
_____
_____
_____
_____
_____
_____
_____
_____
_____
_____
_____
_____
_____
_____
_____

Eastern Equine Encephalitis

Weapon
CDC Bioterrorism Category: B

Alternate Names
EEE

Etiology
Eastern equine encephalitis alphavirus family togaviridae

Transmission
Source:	Mosquitoes, esp *aedes, coquillettidia, culex* species
Entry:	Mosquito bite
Human-to-Human:	No

Predisposing/Comorbid Conditions
NA

Demographics
Location:	Eastern USA, esp around freshwater swamps on Atlantic Coast, Gulf Coast, Great Lakes
Populations:	All in infected areas, esp ages <15 years and >50 years
Calendar:	Year-round

Systems
Nervous

Incubation
3-15 days after mosquito bite

Signs/Symptoms [2]

Abdomen – pain

Body, gen – edema

Bowel movements, control – decreased/absent

Bowel movements – diarrhea

Chills

Consciousness – loss, prolonged (coma)

Cranial nerve VII – palsy

Eyes, motion general – jerky (nystagmus)

Eyes, periorbital – edema

Eyes, vision – light sensitivity, increased (photophobia)

Face – edema

Gait – ataxic

Head – pain (headache)

Joints – pain (arthralgia)

Mentation – confusion

Mentation – delirium

Mentation – feeling of weakness (malaise)

Mood – labile

Mood – lethargic, slowed

Mood – restless, irritable

Muscles, movement – jerks (myoclonus)

Muscles, movement – spontaneous/involuntary

Muscles – pain (myalgia)

Muscles – paralysis [1]

Muscles – weak [1]

Nausea

Neck, post – pain

Neck, post – stiff (meningismus)

Seizures

Sign: Babinski's

Signs/symptoms, nervous system – multiple other

Speech – absent (aphonia) or loss (aphasia)

Temperature, body – elevated (fever)

Tendons, reflexes – decreased

Tendons, reflexes – increased

Throat – sore

Urination, spontaneous control – decreased/absent (urinary incontinence)

Vomiting

Differentiation
Includes, but not limited to:
  Other encephalitides

Complications
  Mild-severe permanent neurologic damage in about 50% of survivors

Laboratory
  Blood IgM-specific antibodies – present
  Blood sodium – decreased [4]
  Blood WBC – increased (leukocytosis)
  CSF IgM-specific antibodies – present
  CSF pressure – increased
  CSF protein – increased
  CSF WBC – increased

ECG
  NA in absence of complications

Imaging
  NA in absence of complications

Other Tests
  NA in absence of complications

Treatment – Nonpharmacologic
  NS

Treatment – Pharmacologic
  NS

Treatment – Surgical/Invasive
  NA

Precautions
  Standard

Primary Prevention

Vaccine: no

Course

33% fatal ☠

Notes

[1] Sudden onset; hemiparesis with tendon reflex asymmetry and positive Babinski sign

[2] Many persons infected with EEE virus have no symptoms or a mild ("flu-like") course without encephalitis symptoms

[3] Most common: VI, VII, XII

[4] Due to inappropriate antidiuretic hormone secretion

http://www.argus1.com/eee

Updates

Ebola Hemorrhagic Fever

Weapon
CDC Bioterrorism Category: A

Alternate Names
African hemorrhagic fever

Etiology
Ebola virus (filovirus)

Primarily infects lymphatic system, testes, ovaries, liver, with secondary severe effects on blood coagulation

Transmission
Source:	Infected human blood, secretions, organs, semen; (?) Monkeys and chimpanzees in/from jungles
Entry:	Contact
	Ingestion
Human-to-Human:	Yes

Predisposing/Comorbid Conditions
NA

Demographics
Location:	Africa, Asia [8]
Populations:	All, esp monkey handlers, laboratory personnel
Calendar:	Year-round

Systems
Coagulation
Gastrointestinal
Nervous
Optic
Skin

Incubation
3-21 days

Signs/Symptoms
Abdomen – pain
Abdomen – tender
Appetite – decreased (anorexia)
Bowel movements – diarrhea
Bowel movements – blood or black (hematochezia) (melena)
Breathing – rapid (tachypnea)
Chest, gen – pain
Chills
Cough, acute NS
Eyes, conjunctivae – injected
Eyes – burning, itching
Head – pain (headache)
Heart rate – increased (tachycardia)
Hiccups [1]
Joints – pain (arthralgia)
Lymph nodes, gen – enlarged (lymphadenopathy)
Mentation – apathy
Mentation – confusion
Mentation – fatigue
Mouth, gingiva – bleeding
Mouth, mucosa – hemorrhage
Mouth, mucosa – ulcers
Muscles – pain (myalgia)
Nausea
Nose – blood (epistaxis)
Skin, color – yellow (jaundice)
Skin – rash, desquamating [2]
Skin – rash, maculopapular [3]
Sputum – blood (hemoptysis)
Swallowing – difficult (dysphagia)
Swallowing – pain (odynophagia)
Temperature, body – elevated (fever)
Throat – sore
Vagina – blood
Vomiting
Vomiting – blood (hematemesis)

Differentiation

Includes, but not limited to:
   Malaria
   Other viral hemorrhagic fevers
   Rickettsial diseases
   Typhoid fever

Complications

Include, but not limited to:
   Abortion
   Blindness
   Disseminated intravascular coagulation (DIC)
   Hepatic failure
   Massive hemorrhage
   Myocarditis
   Orchitis
   Pancreatitis
   Renal failure
   Shock
   Transverse myelitis
   Uveitis

Laboratory [11] ▲

   Blood amylase – increased
   Blood creatinine – increased
   Blood culture – positive
   Blood ELISA IgG antibodies – positive [6]
   Blood liver enzymes – increased
   Blood lymphocytes – decreased (lymphopenia)
   Blood platelets – decreased (thrombocytopenia)
   Blood prothrombin time – increased
   Blood WBC – decreased (leukopenia)
   Blood WBC – left shift [4]
   Semen culture – positive
   Urine protein – present

ECG

   NA in absence of complications [5]

Imaging

NA in absence of complications

Other Tests

NA in absence of complications

Treatment – Nonpharmacologic

NS

Treatment – Pharmacologic

Heparin for DIC
Immune serum transfusion [12]
Replace blood clotting factors

Treatment – Surgical/Invasive

NA in absence of complications

Precautions [11] ▲

Airborne
Avoid direct contact with victim or body secretions [9] ▲

Primary Prevention

Vaccine: in development
Barrier techniques ▲
Disposal of infected human fluids ▲
Quarantine and handling of monkeys from Africa ▲

Course

20-90% fatal ☠

Notes

[1]   Esp fatal cases
[2]   About day 5
[3]   Esp trunk, back
[4]   Early in course
[5]   I.e., myocarditis
[6]   Week 2
[7]   Through contact with infected blood, organs, secretions, semen

[8]   And any location of imported monkeys from Sub-Saharan Africa
[9]   Highly contagious ▲
[10]   Due to shock and multi-organ failure
[11]   BSL-4 procedures
[12]   Efficacy uncertain

http://www.argus1.com/?ebola

Updates

_____
_____
_____
_____
_____
_____
_____
_____
_____
_____
_____
_____
_____
_____
_____
_____
_____
_____
_____

Epsilon Toxin – *Clostridia Perfringens*

Note: there is no available documentation on the effect of epsilon toxin on humans. It is produced by type b and type d strains of C. perfringens, which uncommonly infect humans, but can cause disease in animals; this is the basis for concern that this substance could be used as a bio-chemical weapon involving the body systems listed. ▲

Weapon
CDC Bioterrorism Category: B

Alternate Names
NA

Etiology
Epsilon toxin of *C perfringens*

Transmission
Source: Uncertain
Entry: Uncertain
Human-to-Human: No

Predisposing/Comorbid Conditions
NA

Demographics
Location: NA
Populations: All
Calendar: NA

Systems [1]
Gastrointestinal

Nervous
Respiratory – lower

Time to Clinical Onset
ND

Signs/Symptoms
ND

Differentiation
ND

Complications
ND

Laboratory
ND

Imaging
ND

Other Tests
ND

Treatment – Nonpharmacologic
ND

Treatment – Pharmacologic
ND

Treatment – Surgical/Invasive
ND

Precautions
ND

Primary prevention
ND

Course
ND

Note
[1] Presumed, based on animal studies

http://www.argus1.com/?epsilonclostridia

Updates

_____
_____
_____
_____
_____
_____
_____
_____
_____
_____
_____
_____
_____
_____
_____
_____
_____
_____
_____
_____

Giardiasis

Weapon
No

Alternate Names
Giardia enteritis
Lambliasis

Etiology
Giardia lamblia (*G intestinalis*)

Transmission
Source:	Contaminated water, uncooked food, and other sources contaminated by infected human and animal excreta [7]
Entry:	Ingestion
Human-to-Human:	Yes (fecal-oral)

Predisposing/Comorbid Conditions
Decreased gastric acidity
Immune deficiency
Prior gastric surgery

Demographics
Location:	Global
Populations:	All
Calendar:	Year-round

Systems
Gastrointestinal

Incubation
7-14 days

Signs/Symptoms [3]

Abdomen – cramps
Abdomen – flatulence
Abdomen – fullness
Abdomen – pain
Appearance, gen – wasting (cachexia)
Appetite – reduced (anorexia)
Bowel movements, stool – fatty (steatorrhea) [2]
Bowel movements – constipation [10]
Bowel movements – diarrhea [1]
Joints – pain (arthralgia) [6]
Mentation – fatigue
Mentation – weakness (malaise)
Nausea
Skin – rash, itching (urticaria) [10]
Temperature, body – increased (fever) [10]
Vomiting
Weight – loss

Differentiation

Includes, but not limited to:
Other causes of gastroenteritis

Complications

Include, but not limited to:
Dehydration
Vitamin malabsorption

Laboratory

Blood ELISA assay – positive
Stool cysts – positive [4]

ECG

NA in absence of complications

Imaging

NA in absence of complications

Other Tests

Duodenal aspiration and biopsy

Treatment – Nonpharmacologic
Fluids and electrolytes

Treatment – Pharmacologic [5]
Albendazole
Furazolidone
Metronidazole
Nitazoxanide
Paromomycin
Quinacrine
Tinidazole

Treatment – Surgical/Invasive
NA in absence of complications

Precautions
Enteric [8] ▲

Primary Prevention
Avoid contaminated sources
Standard

Course [9]
Variable duration – weeks to months
Rarely fatal

Notes
[1]   Often explosive, watery
[2]   Stools greasy, foul-smelling
[3]   Most infected persons have no symptoms
[4]   May be missed due to intermittent shedding, requiring multiple samples until positive; stools negative for blood, pus, mucous
[5]   Reduces symptoms and prevents infection spread
[6]   Reactive arthritis – uncommon
[7]   Cysts remain viable outside host for long periods in water and uncooked food
[8]   Strict handwashing and other techniques around infected persons ▲
[9]   May recur after full therapeutic course
[10]   Uncommon

http://www.argus1.com/?giardia

Updates

_____

_____

_____

_____

_____

_____

_____

_____

_____

_____

_____

_____

_____

_____

_____

_____

_____

_____

Glanders

Weapon
CDC Bioterrorism Category: B

Alternate Names
Farcy [2]

Etiology
Burkholderia mallei (*pseudomonas mallei*) [4]

Transmission
Source:	Equids (horses, mules, donkeys), goats, dogs, cats
Entry:	Contact
	Inhalation
Human-to-Human:	Yes

Predisposing/Comorbid Conditions
Broken skin

Demographic
Locations:	Global [3]
Populations:	Veterinarians, horse handlers, laboratory personnel, butchers
Calendar:	Year-round

Systems
Lymphatic
Musculoskeletal
Oropharynx
Skin

Incubation

1-5 days

Signs/Symptoms

Abdomen – pain
Appetite – decreased (anorexia)
Bowel movements – diarrhea
Breathing – difficult (dyspnea)
Chest – pain, pleuritic
Chills
Cough – acute, NS
Eyes, light sensitivity – increased (photophobia)
Eyes, tears (lacrimation) – increased
Head – pain (headache)
Lymph nodes, neck – enlarged
Lymph nodes, regional – enlarged
Mentation – confusion
Mentation – weakness (malaise)
Mouth, mucosa – ulcers
Muscles – abscess
Muscles – pain (myalgia)
Nose, drainage – increased (rhinorrhea, coryza)
Nose, mucosa – ulcers
Skin – nodule [1, 2]
Skin – rash, papular [2]
Skin – rash, pustular [2]
Skin – ulcer, single [2]
Spleen – enlarged (splenomegaly)
Sweating – nocturnal (night sweats)
Temperature, body – elevated (fever)
Throat – sore

Differentiation

Includes, but not limited to:
All other causes of pneumonia
All other septicemias
All other skin infections

Complications

Include, but not limited to:
Brain abscess
Liver abscess
Orchitis
Osteomyelitis
Meningitis
Pneumonia
Spleen abscess

Laboratory [5] ▲

Blood culture – positive
Blood lymphocytes – increased (lymphocytosis)
Blood serology – positive
Blood WBC – increased (leukocytosis)
Skin culture – positive
Sputum culture – positive
Urine culture – positive

ECG

NS in absence of complications

Imaging

Pneumonia
Lungs – cavitations
Lungs – infiltrates, bilat
Lungs – nodules, miliary

Other Tests

NS in absence of complications

Treatment – Nonpharmacologic

NS

Treatment – Pharmacologic [6]

Antibiotics
Amoxicillin
Ceftazidime
Ceftriaxone

Doxycycline
Gentamycin
Trimethoprim – sulfa

Treatment – Surgical/Invasive
Abscess drainage

Precautions
Handling specimens [5] ▲

Primary Prevention
Vaccine: no
Animal control
Prophylactic antibiotic with exposure [7]

Course
Untreated mortality almost 100% ☠

Notes
[1] With nodular lymphangitic cord extending to regional lymph nodes
[2] Termed "farcy" when localized to skin
[3] Eradicated in most areas of world, except Africa
[4] Gram neg aerobe
[5] BSL-3 procedures; agent is highly infectious with exposure to only a few organisms ▲
[6] Relative efficacies uncertain; protocols vary according to infection site and whether local or systemic
[7] Efficacy uncertain

http://www.argus1.com/?glanders

Updates

_____
_____
_____
_____
_____
_____
_____
_____
_____
_____
_____
_____
_____
_____
_____
_____
_____
_____
_____
_____
_____

Hantavirus Pulmonary Syndrome

Weapon
CDC Bioterrorism Category: C

Alternate Names
HPS

Etiology
Hantavirus, family Bunyaviridiae

Pulmonary vascular endothelial damage with fluid extravasation and necrosis of surrounding tissue

Transmission
Source:	Rodent excreta or saliva
Entry:	Skin contact
	Inhalation
Human-to-Human:	No

Predisposing/Comorbid Conditions
Broken skin

Demographics
Locations:	Europe, Asia, N America
Populations:	All, esp Native Americans, hikers, campers
Calendar:	Year-round, esp autumn

Systems
Respiratory – lower

Incubation
1-5 weeks

Signs/Symptoms
Abdomen – pain
Appetite – decreased (anorexia)
Arterial pressure – decreased (hypotension) [7]
Breathing – difficult, rest (rest dyspnea)
Breathing – rapid (tachypnea)
Chest – rales
Chest – tightness
Chills
Cough – acute NS
Dizziness (lightheaded)
Mentation – fatigue
Head – pain (headache)
Heart rate – rapid (tachycardia)
Joints – pain (arthralgia)
Muscles – pain (myalgia) [2]
Nausea
Spleen – enlarged (splenomegaly)
Temperature, body – elevated (fever)
Vomiting

Differentiation
Includes, but not limited to:
Acute respiratory distress syndrome (ARDS)
Congestive heart failure
Influenza
Other causes of pulmonary edema
Pneumonia

Complications
Include, but not limited to:
Noncardiac pulmonary edema
Respiratory failure
Shock

Laboratory [4] ▲
Blood arterial pO_2 – decreased (hypoxia)
Blood creatinine – increased [3]
Blood creatine kinase – increased

Blood ELISA antibodies – positive
Blood Hgb, Hct – increased [5]
Blood LDH – increased [8]
Blood liver enzymes – increased
Blood lymphocytes – atypical
Blood platelets – decreased (thrombocytopenia) [1]
Blood prothrombin time – increased [1]
Blood PTT – increased [1]
Blood urea nitrogen – increased [3]
Blood WBC – increased (leukocytosis)
Blood WBC – left shift
Urine protein – present (proteinuria)

ECG
NS abnormalities

Imaging
Lungs, interstitium – edema (Kerley B lines)
Lungs, parenchyma general – infiltrates
Lungs, pleura – fluid (pleural effusion)
Lungs, vasculature – congested

Other Tests
NA in absence of complications

Treatment – Nonpharmacologic
Fluid replacement [6] ▲
Mechanical ventilation
Oxygen [10]
Volume replacement

Treatment – Pharmacologic
Ribivarin [9]

Treatment – Surgical/Invasive
NA in absence of complications

Precautions
BSL-4 procedures ▲

Primary Prevention
Vaccine: investigational
Rodent control

Course

Untreated
Up to 50% mortality ☠

Notes
[1]   Hemorrhagic manifestations as in hemorrhagic fever with renal syndrome absent
[2]   Esp large muscle groups, i.e., thighs, hips, back, shoulders
[3]   Mild
[4]   BSL-4 procedures ▲
[5]   Due to hemoconcentration from fluid extravasation into lungs
[6]   Administer with caution to avoid pulmonary edema
[7]   1/3 of cases
[8]   May be greatly elevated
[9]   Uncertain efficacy for this condition
[10]   Extracorporeal membrane oxygenation may be needed

http://www.argus1.com/?hanta

Updates

_____
_____
_____
_____
_____
_____
_____
_____
_____
_____
_____
_____
_____
_____
_____

Hemorrhagic Fever with Renal Syndrome

Weapon
CDC Bioterrorism Category: C

Alternate Names
Epidemic hemorrhagic fever
Hemorrhagic nephrosonephritis
HFRS
Korean hemorrhagic fever
Nephropathica epidemica

Etiology
Virus of genus *hantavirus*

Vascular endothelial damage and hemorrhagic necrosis of adrenal medulla, anterior pituitary, right atrium; retroperitoneal gelatinous edema

Transmission
Source:	Rodents
Entry:	Contact
	Inhalation
Human-to-Human:	No

Predisposing/Comorbid Conditions
NA

Demographics
Location:	Europe, Asia
Populations:	All, esp persons engaged in outdoor activities (soldiers, farmers, campers, etc)
Calendar:	Year-round

Systems
Cardiovascular
Coagulation
Renal/Genitourinary

Incubation
2-40 days (average 2 weeks)

Signs/Symptoms
Abdomen – pain [1]
Appetite – decreased (anorexia)
Arterial press – elevated [5, 7]
Arterial press – low [2, 6] ▲
Back – pain
Chills
Cough – acute NS
Dizziness (lightheaded)
Eyes, conjunctivae – injected
Eyes, periorbital – edema
Eyes, vision – blurred
Head – pain (headache)
Heart rate – rapid (tachycardia)
Mentation – fatigue
Mentation – nonspecific changes
Mentation – weakness (malaise)
Mouth, palate – injected
Mouth, palate – petechiae
Muscles – pain (myalgia) [4]
Nausea
Skin, axillae – petechiae
Skin, face – flushed [3]
Skin, upper body – flushed, erythematous [3]
Skin – temperature, cool [2]
Spleen – enlarged (splenomegaly)
Temperature, body – elevated (fever)
Throat – injected
Urine volume – decreased (oliguria) [2, 5]
Urine volume – increased (diuresis) [6]
Vomiting

Differentiation

Includes, but not limited to:

    Acute abdomen

    Leptospirosis

    Meningococcemia

    Other causes of renal failure

    Poststreptococcal nephritis

    Rickettsial infection

Complications

Include, but not limited to:

    Noncardiac pulmonary edema

    Shock

Laboratory [9] ▲

    Blood concentration – increased (hemoconcentration)

    Blood creatinine – increased

    Blood electrolytes – abnormal

    Blood IgG-specific antibodies – present

    Blood IgM-specific antibodies – present

    Blood lymphocytes – atypical

    Blood platelets – decreased (thrombocytopenia)

    Blood urea nitrogen (BUN) – increased

    Blood WBC – increased (leukocytosis)

    Blood WBC – left shift

    Urine protein – present

ECG

    Dysrhythmias – atrial [8]

    P wave – abnormal [8]

Imaging

    NA in absence of complications

Other Tests

    NA in absence of complications

Treatment – Nonpharmacologic

    Fluids and electrolytes

Treatment – Pharmacologic
Ribavirin

Treatment – Surgical/Invasive
Dialysis [5]

Precautions
BSL-4 procedures ▲

Primary Prevention
Vaccine: experimental
Rodent control

Course
Mortality up to 5% ☠

Notes
[1]   May resemble acute abdomen
[2]   BP fall may occur abruptly, about 1 week after onset ▲
[3]   Extends to neck, shoulders, upper thorax; blanches with pressure
[4]   Esp large muscles – thighs, hips, back
[5]   Oliguric phase
[6]   Diuretic phase
[7]   May occur suddenly
[8]   Due to right atrial necrosis
[9]   BSL-4 procedures ▲

http://www.argus1.com/?hemren

Updates

_____
_____
_____
_____
_____
_____
_____
_____
_____
_____
_____

Infectious Hepatitis – Acute

Weapon
No

Alternate Names
Viral hepatitis

Etiology
Hepatitis viruses A-E

Transmission
Source:	Blood
	Body fluids
	Excrement
Entry [10]:	Ingestion
	Maternal – fetal
	Parenteral
	Sexual contact
Human-to-Human:	Yes

Predisposing/Comorbid Conditions
Varies with type and includes HIV and pregnancy

Demographics
Location:	Global
Populations:	All, esp IV drug users, persons with multiple sex partners, daycare children, and healthcare workers
Calendar:	Year-round

Systems
Liver/Biliary tract/Pancreas

Incubation

2 weeks – 6 months depending on agent

Signs/Symptoms [1, 2]

Abdomen – pain
Abdomen – tender
Appetite – reduced (anorexia)
Bowel movements – constipation
Bowel movements – diarrhea
Chills
Cough – nonproductive [3]
Eyes, conjunctivae – yellow
Eyes, vision – light sensitivity, increased (photophobia) [3]
Fatigue
Head – pain (headache)
Joints – pain (arthralgia)
Liver – enlarged (hepatomegaly)
Mentation – weakness (malaise)
Muscles – pain (myalgia)
Nausea
Nose – drainage (rhinorrhea, coryza) [3]
Sense of taste – decreased [9]
Skin, color – yellow (jaundice)
Skin – itching (pruritus)
Skin – rash, papular
Skin – rash, pruritic
Skin – rash, vesicular
Spleen – enlarged (splenomegaly)
Stools – light
Temperature, body – elevated (fever) [4]
Throat – sore [3]
Urine – dark
Vomiting

Differentiation

Includes, but not limited to:
Acute fatty liver of pregnancy
Bile duct obstruction
Budd-Chiari syndrome
Drug-induced hepatitis

Hellp syndrome [5]
Immunologic disorders
Influenza (early stage)
Ischemic hepatitis
Other causes of jaundice
Other causes of liver failure
Other liver infections [6]
Wilson's disease

Complications

Include, but not limited to:
Acute liver failure
Aseptic meningoencephalitis
Cholestatic liver injury
Chronic liver failure
Liver carcinoma
Liver cirrhosis

Laboratory

Blood albumin – decreased
Blood bilirubin – increased
Blood IgG-specific antibodies – present
Blood IgM-specific antibodies – present
Blood liver enzymes – increased
Blood prothrombin time – increased

ECG

NA in absence of complications

Imaging

NA in absence of complications

Other Tests

Liver biopsy

Treatment – Nonpharmacologic

Avoid alcohol in acute phase
NS

Treatment – Pharmacologic [7] ▲

NS

Treatment – Surgical/Invasive

Liver transplant for rare cases of liver failure

Precautions [8]

Enteric

Proper disposal/sterilization of parenteral instruments

Primary Prevention

Vaccine: Hepatitis A, B

Avoidance of infected blood and other body fluids [11] ▲

Course

Variable with type and comorbid conditions

Recovery usual

Notes

[1]   Many cases asymptomatic, with liver enzyme rise only manifestation

[2]   In acute phase, all hepatitis types are similar in clinical manifestations

[3]   Initial symptoms "flu-like," last a few days

[4]   Usually low-grade

[5]   "Hemolysis, elevated liver enzymes, low platelets" syndrome; a pregnancy complication

[6]   Brucellosis, cytomegalovirus, Ebstein-Barr (infectious mononucleosis), HIV, leptospirosis, Lyme disease, Q fever, syphilis, yellow fever

[7]   Discontinue and avoid drugs except as necessary during acute phase, esp narcotics and hypnotics ▲

[8]   Pending identification of type; thereafter dictated by transmission routes for specific infecting agent

[9]   Food, cigarettes

[10] Varies with type of hepatitis

[11] Includes screening for infected blood and blood products prior to transfusion ▲

http://www.argus1.com/?hepatitisacute

Updates

_____
_____
_____
_____
_____
_____
_____
_____
_____

Infectious Mononucleosis

Weapon
No

Alternate Names
Glandular fever
Kissing disease
Mono
Monocytic angina
Pfeiffer's disease

Etiology
Ebstein-Barr virus (EBV)

Transmission
Source:	Human saliva
Transmission:	Ingestion
	Blood transfusion
Human-to-human:	Yes

Predisposing/Comorbid Conditions
NA

Demographics
Location:	Global
Populations:	All [10]
Calendar:	Year-round

Systems
Liver/Biliary tract/Pancreas
Lymphatic
Oropharynx

Incubation
4-6 weeks

Signs/Symptoms [12]

Abdomen, LUQ – pain [3]
Abdomen, LUQ – tenderness [3]
Abdomen – pain [11] ▲
Appetite – decreased (anorexia)
Eyes, lids – swollen (edema)
Head – pain (headache)
Liver – enlarged (hepatomegaly) [4]
Lymph nodes, epitrochlear – enlarged [7]
Lymph nodes, gen – enlarged [5]
Lymph nodes, post cervical – enlarged [7]
Lymph nodes, tonsillar – enlarged
Lymph nodes, tonsillar – exudate
Mentation – fatigue
Mentation – weakness (malaise)
Mouth, palate – petechiae [8]
Muscles – pain (myalgia)
Nausea
Skin – rash, macular/papular [9]
Spleen – enlarged (splenomegaly) [6, 11] ▲
Spleen – tender [11] ▲
Temperature, body – elevated (fever)
Throat – exudate
Throat – injected
Throat – sore

Differentiation

Includes, but not limited to:
Lymphocytic leukemia
Other forms of hepatitis
Streptococcal pharyngitis

Complications

Include, but not limited to:
Airway impairment
Encephalitis
Gullain-Barré syndrome
Hemolytic anemia

Interstitial pneumonia
Meningitis
Myocarditis
Orchitis
Pancreatitis
Parotitis
Pericarditis
Reye's syndrome
Spleen rupture
Transverse myelitis

Laboratory

Blood alkaline phosphatase – increased
Blood bilirubin – increased
Blood EBV-specific antibodies – positive
Blood heterophile antibody – positive
Blood liver enzymes – increased
Blood lymphocytes – atypical [1]
Blood lymphocytes – increased (lymphocytosis)
Blood platelets – decreased (thrombocytopenia) [2]
Blood WBC – decreased (leukopenia)

ECG

NA in absence of complications, esp myocarditis/pericarditis

Imaging

NA in absence of complications

Other Tests

NA in absence of complications

Treatment – Nonpharmacologic

Avoid trauma to spleen
Bed rest – acute phase

Treatment – Pharmacologic

Corticosteroids for airway impairment and other complications

Treatment – Surgical/Invasive

Surgery for spleen rupture

Precautions
Standard

Primary Prevention
Vaccine: no

Course
Usual resolution – 1-4 weeks

Notes
[1]   Antigenically altered T lymphocytes; also found in cytomegalovirus infection, drug reactions, herpes virus, malaria, mumps, mycoplasma, rubella, rubeola, serum sickness, toxoplasmosis, tuberculosis, typhoid, viral hepatitis

[2]   Mild, seldom clinically significant

[3]   Due to splenic enlargement; may be presenting complaint

[4]   10%

[5]   90%

[6]   50%

[7]   Differentiation from other causes of lymphadenopathy

[8]   Esp at hard-soft palate junction

[9]   May be precipitated by ampicillin or amoxicillin

[10]   Esp severe in older persons and in immune compromise

[11]   Palpate abdomen carefully to avoid spleen rupture ▲

[12]   May be asymptomatic, esp young children

http://www.argus1.com/?infmono

Updates

Influenza

Weapon
No

Alternate Names
Flu
Grippe

Etiology
Influenza virus (types A,B,C)

Causes intracelluar viral replication in upper and lower respiratory tract within 24 hours after infection; present in secretions for 3-5 days; edema and hyperemia of upper and lower respiratory cells, esp bronchial epithelial cells, with loss of cilia; extends to pulmonary alveolar cells in pneumonia

Transmission
Source: Human and nonhuman animals
Entry: Inhalation
                     Contact
Human-to-Human: Yes

Predisposing/Comorbid Conditions
Chronic obstructive pulmonary disease
Heart disease
Third-trimester pregnancy

Demographic
Locations: Global
Populations: All, esp severe in infants and aged
Calendar: Year-round, with regional variations including winter month increase in northern latitudes

Systems

Gastrointestinal
Musculoskeletal
Optic
Oropharynx
Respiratory – upper

Incubation

1-5 days

Signs/Symptoms [8]

Abdomen – pain [5]
Appetite – decreased (anorexia)
Bowel movements – diarrhea
Chest, ant – pain, pleuritic
Chills
Cough – nonproductive
Cough – productive
Dizziness (lightheaded)
Eyes, conjunctivae – injected
Eyes, light sensitivity – increased (photophobia)
Eyes, motion – painful
Eyes, tears (lacrimation) – increased
Face, parotid glands – enlarged [1]
Face – flushed
Head – pain (headache)
Joints – pain (arthralgia)
Lymph nodes, ant cervical – enlarged
Mentation – fatigue
Mentation – weakness (malaise)
Muscles – pain (myalgia)
Muscles – stiff
Muscles – tender
Nausea
Nose, drainage – increased (rhinorrhea, coryza)
Nose, mucosa – inflamed
Nose – congested
Temperature, body – elevated (fever)
Throat – dry
Throat – injected

Throat – sore
Voice – hoarse
Vomiting

Differentiation

Resembles numerous other viral and bacterial infectious diseases in early stages, i.e., malaise, headache, fever, myalgia, sore throat

Complications

Include, but not limited to:

Acute bronchitis
Asthma exacerbation
Croup
Cystic fibrosis exacerbation
Encephalopathy
Myelitis
Myocarditis
Myositis
Pericarditis
Pneumonia – bacterial
Pneumonia – viral
Radiculopathy – Guillain-Barré type
Reye's syndrome [6] ▲
Rhabdomyolysis
Toxic shock syndrome

Laboratory

Blood arterial pH – decreased (acidosis) [2]
Blood concentration – increased [2]
Respiratory secretion rapid antigen test – positive, type A, B

ECG

NA in absence of complications [4]

Imaging

NA in absence of pneumonia or other complications

Other Tests

NA in absence of complications

Treatment – Nonpharmacologic

Fluids and electrolytes

Treatment – Pharmacologic [7]
Symptomatic only [9] ▲

Treatment – Surgical/Invasive
NA in absence of complications

Precautions
Standard

Primary Prevention
Vaccine: yes

Course
Severity and duration may be ameliorated by amantadine in some
cases of type A [7]
Usual duration – 3-5 days

Notes
[1] Other salivary glands may also be enlarged
[2] Due to dehydration
[3] Esp valvular disease and congestive heart failure
[4] I.e., myocarditis and pericarditis
[5] May be local or diffuse
[6] Usually with aspirin ▲
[7] Consult current guidelines for use of antiviral agents
[8] Symptom onset typically sudden
[9] Avoid aspirin and aspirin-containing products for febrile infections in
children <19 years due to association with Reye's syndrome ▲

http://www.argus1.com/?influ

Updates

_____
_____
_____
_____
_____
_____
_____
_____
_____
_____
_____

Lassa Fever

Weapon
CDC Bioterrorism Category: A

Alternate Names
NA

Etiology
Lassa virus (arenavirus)

Endothelial cell damage, platelet dysfunction, myocardial suppression, release of cytokines and other mediators of shock/inflammation

Transmission
Source:	Rodent (rat *mastomys nataensis*) excreta/direct contact
Entry:	Contact
	Ingestion
	Inhalation
	Sexual
Human-to-Human:	Yes

Predisposing/Comorbid Conditions
Pregnancy [3, 4] ▲

Demographics
Location:	West Africa
Populations:	All
Calendar:	Year-round

Systems
Cardiovascular
Coagulation

Gastrointestinal
Lymphatic
Musculoskeletal
Nervous
Oropharynx
Otic
Skin

Incubation

1-3 weeks

Signs/Symptoms [10]

Abdomen, epigastrium – pain
Abdomen, lower – pain
Abdomen – tender
Arterial pressure – decreased (hypotension)
Back – pain
Bowel movements – diarrhea
Bowel movements – blood or black (hematochezia) (melena)
Chest, ant – pain, nonpleuritic rest
Cough – nonproductive
Cranial nerve VIII – palsy
Dizziness (lightheaded)
Ears, hearing – loss (deafness) [1]
Ears – ringing (tinnitus)
Eyes, conjunctivae – hemorrhage
Eyes, conjunctivae – injected
Face – edema
Hair, head – loss (alopecia)
Head, frontal – pain
Head – pain (headache)
Heart – friction rub, pericardial
Heart rate – decreased relative to fever (relative bradycardia)
Joints, gen – pain (arthralgia)
Lungs – friction rub, pleural
Lymph nodes – enlarged
Mentation – confusion
Mentation – weakness (malaise)
Mouth, gingiva – bleeding

Mouth, mucosa – ulcers
Muscles, movement – incoordinated (ataxia)
Muscles – pain (myalgia)
Muscles – tender
Muscles – tremors, rest
Nausea
Neck – edema
Nose – blood (epistaxis)
Seizures
Skin – rash, macular/papular
Temperature, body – elevated (fever)
Throat – exudate
Throat – sore
Throat – ulcers
Throat – vesicles
Vagina – blood
Vomiting
Vomiting – blood (hematemesis)

Differentiation

Includes, but not limited to:
Anicteric hepatitis
Arboviral infection
Bacterial or viral conjunctivitis
Bacterial sepsis
Enterovirus infection
Leptospirosis
Malaria
Meningitis
Other hemorrhagic fevers
Typhoid fever

Complications

Include, but not limited to:
Abortion [3, 4] ▲
Deafness [12]
Encephalitis
Myocarditis
Occulogyric crisis

Orchitis
Pericarditis
Systemic capillary "leak" syndrome [11]

Laboratory [7] ▲

Blood culture – positive
Blood liver enzymes – increased
Blood serology – positive (rise in titer) [13]
Blood WBC – decreased (leukopenia)
Throat culture – positive
Urine protein – present (heavy)(proteinuria)

ECG

NS abnormalities [8]

Imaging

Lungs – NS abnormalities

Other Tests

NA in absence of complications [9]

Treatment – Nonpharmacologic

Fluids and electrolytes

Treatment – Pharmacologic

Ribavirin [2]

Treatment – Surgical/Invasive

NA in absence of complications

Precautions

BSL-4 procedures ▲
Standard

Primary Prevention

Vaccine: no
Contact surveillance [6]
Isolation of patients
Rodent control

Course

Hospitalized case mortality 15-20% [5] ☠

Notes

[1] Sensorineural; up to 33%; appears in early convalescence; unilateral or bilateral; deafness may be permanent

[2] Begin in first 6 days for optimum effect

[3] Third-trimester mortality >30% ☠

[4] "Swollen baby syndrome"; fetal and neonatal mortality >85% ☠

[5] Poor prognostic signs: high viremia, serum aspartate aminotransferase >150 iu/l, bleeding, edema, encephalitis, third trimester of pregnancy

[6] WHO: body temp checks 2x/day for 3 weeks after last exposure

[7] BSL-4 procedures ▲

[8] Due to myocarditis

[9] I.e., pleural effusion, infiltrates

[10] Many cases asymptomatic or mild

[11] Includes hypotension, ascites, pleural effusion, peripheral vasoconstriction

[12] Unilateral or bilateral, transient or permanent

[13] Correlates with prognosis

http://www.argus1.com/?lassa

Updates

_____
_____
_____
_____
_____
_____
_____
_____
_____
_____
_____
_____
_____
_____
_____
_____

Legionellosis

Weapon
No

Alternate Names
Legionnaires' disease [5]
Pontiac fever [6]

Etiology
Legionella pneumophilia [16]

Transmision
Source:	Contaminated water, including cooling towers, showers, faucets, spas, hot tubs
Entry:	Inhalation [17]
Human-to-Human:	No

Predisposing/Comorbid Conditions
Advanced age
Cigarette smoking
Cancer
COPD
Diabetes mellitus
Immune deficiency
Organ transplant
Renal disease

Demographics
Location:	Global
Populations:	All, increases with age
Calendar:	Year-round [15]

Systems
Gastrointestinal
Nervous
Respiratory – lower

Incubation

2-10 days

Signs/Symptoms

Abdomen – tender [11]
Abdomen – pain
Appetite – decreased (anorexia)
Bowel movements – diarrhea [9]
Breath sounds, local – decreased
Breath sounds – crackling (rales)
Breathing – difficult, rest (rest dyspnea)
Chest, gen – pain, pleuritic
Chest, local – consolidation signs
Chest, local – pain, pleuritic
Chills
Cough – acute NS
Cough – nonproductive [2]
Cough – productive
Head – pain (headache) [10]
Heart rate – decreased relative to fever (relative bradycardia)
Liver – enlarged (hepatomegaly) [11]
Mentation – confusion
Mentation – fatigue
Mentation – hallucinations
Mentation – sleepy (somnolence)
Mentation – weakness (malaise)
Mood – depression
Mood – lethargy
Muscles – pain (myalgia)
Muscles – weakness
Nausea
Neurologic changes, focal [12]
Seizures
Spleen – enlarged (splenomegaly) [12]
Sputum – blood (hemoptysis) [3]
Sputum – clear
Sputum – purulent
Temperature, body – increased (fever) [8]
Vomiting

Differentiation
Includes, but not limited to:
Acute abdomen
Gastroenteritis
Influenza
Metastatic infection [19]
Other forms of pneumonia [18]
Pancreatitis

Complications [4]
Include, but not limited to:
Bowel abscess
Cellulitis
Disseminated intravascular coagulation (DIC)
Myocarditis
Pancreatitis
Pericarditis
Peritonitis
Postcardiotomy syndrome
Prosthetic valve endocarditis
Pyelonephritis
Sinusitis

Laboratory
Blood bilirubin – increased
Blood cold agglutinins – present
Blood creatine kinase – increased
Blood creatinine – increased [13]
Blood culture – positive
Blood liver enzymes – increased
Blood platelets – decreased (thrombocytopenia) [13]
Blood phosphate – decreased
Blood sodium – decreased
Blood WBC – decreased (leukopenia) [13]
Blood WBC – increased (leukocytosis)
Pleural fluid culture – positive
Sputum culture – positive
Urine antigen – positive
Urine myoglobin – positive (myoglobinuria)
Urine protein – present (proteinuria)

Urine RBC – present (hematuria, microhematuria)
Urine WBC – present (pyuria)

ECG
NA in absence of complications [14]

Imaging
Lungs, parenchyma – cavitation
Lungs, parenchyma – consolidation
Lungs, parenchyma – infiltrates [7]
Lungs, pleura – fluid (effusion)

Other Tests
NA in absence of complications

Treatment – Nonpharmacologic
NS

Treatment – Pharmacologic
Antibiotics
    Macrolides
    Quinolones
    Tetracyclines

Treatment – Surgical/Invasive
NA in absence of complications

Precautions
Standard

Primary Prevention
Water system control [20]

Course
Legionnaires' form – 10-15% mortality ☠

Notes
[1]   For "Legionnaires' pneumonia"
[2]   Initially

[3]   Scanty, up to 1/3 of cases

[4]   Sometimes via bacteremic dissemination from primary pulmonary site

[5]   More severe form, includes pneumonia

[6]   Mild form

[7]   Unilateral early, bilateral later

[8]   Up to 105°F

[9]   Typically watery

[10]   Early in course

[11]   Usually mild

[12]   Uncommon

[13]   Severe cases

[14]   Abnormal in myocarditis, pericarditis

[15]   Sporadic and epidemic forms

[16]   Multiply within many types of amebae in water

[17]   Aerosolized contaminated water

[18]   Closely resembles pneumococcal pneumonia

[19]   Brain, muscle, etc; rare except in immune compromised patients

[20]   Esp cooling towers

http://www.argus1.com/?legion

Updates

_____

_____

_____

_____

_____

_____

_____

_____

_____

_____

_____

_____

_____

_____

_____

Leptospirosis

Weapon
No

Alternate Names
Canicola fever
Hemorrhagic jaundice
Mud fever
Swineherd disease
Weil's disease [1]

Etiology
Genus *leptospira*

Disseminates from entry point via bloodstream to organs, esp kidneys (interstitial nephritis), liver (centrilobular necrosis), and muscle (focal necrosis)

Transmission

Source:	Water, food and soil contaminated by urine from infected animals, including rats, raccoons, dogs, pigs, cattle, deer
Entry:	Skin/mucous membranes
	Ingestion
	Inhalation
Human-to-Human:	Rare

Predisposing/Comorbid Conditions
Skin abrasion

Demographic

Location:	Global [11]
Population:	All, esp farmers, sewer workers, recreational swimmers, veterinarians
Calendar:	Year-round, with late summer peak, esp after periods of increased rainfall

Systems
Cardiovascular
Coagulation
Liver/Biliary tract/Pancreas
Musculoskeletal
Nervous
Optic
Renal/Genitourinary
Skin

Incubation
7-14 days

Signs/Symptoms [2]
Abdomen, RUQ – tender
Abdomen – pain
Appetite – decreased (anorexia)
Back, lumbar – pain
Bone – pain
Bowel movements – diarrhea
Breath sounds – crackling (rales)
Chest – pain, pleuritic
Chills
Cough – acute NS
Eyes, conjunctivae – hemorrhage [3]
Eyes, conjunctivae – injected [3]
Eyes, light sensitivity – increased (photophobia)
Head – pain (headache) [4]
Heart rate – decreased relative to fever (relative bradycardia)
Joints – pain (arthralgia)
Legs, walking – pain
Liver – enlarged (hepatomegaly)
Lymph nodes – enlarged
Mentation – confused
Mentation – nonspecific changes
Muscles – pain (myalgia) [5]
Muscles – rigid
Muscles – tender
Nausea
Neck, post – pain [6]

Neck, post – stiff [6]
Skin, color – yellow (jaundice)
Skin, sensation – increased (hyperesthesia, causalgia)
Skin – rash, itching (urticaria) [7]
Skin – rash, macular [7]
Skin – rash, petechiae [7]
Spleen – enlarged (splenomegaly) [8]
Sputum – blood (hemoptysis) [9]
Temperature, body – elevated (fever)
Throat – injected
Throat – sore
Urine – blood (hematuria)
Urine – cloudy
Vomiting

Differentiation

Includes, but not limited to:
Acute cholecystitis
Encephalitis
Hepatitis
Influenza
Meningitis
Renal failure

Complications

Include, but not limited to:
Abortion
Acute respiratory distress syndrome (ARDS)
Arthritis
Cardiac dysrhythmias
Congestive heart failure
Disseminated intravascular coagulation
Guillain-Barré syndrome
Hemorrhage – adrenal
Hemorrhage – gastrointestinal
Hemorrhage – pulmonary
Hemorrhage – subarachnoid
Liver failure
Meningoencephalitis – aseptic
Myocarditis [12]

Pericarditis
Pulmonary failure
Renal failure
Rhabdomyolysis
Transverse myelitis
Uveitis

Laboratory
Blood alkaline phosphatase – increased
Blood bilirubin – increased
Blood culture – positive
Blood Hgb/Hct – decreased (anemia)
Blood liver enzymes – increased
Blood platelets – decreased (thrombocytopenia)
Blood prothrombin time – increased
Blood serology – positive
Blood urea nitrogen – increased
Blood WBC – increased (leukocytosis)
CSF culture – positive
CSF protein – increased
Urine casts, hyaline – present
Urine culture – positive
Urine protein – present (proteinuria)
Urine RBC – present (hematuria)
Urine WBC – present (pyuria)

ECG
Dysrhythmias, atrial and ventricular
Rate – slow relative to temperature (relative bradycardia)

Imaging
Lungs – infiltrates

Other Tests
NA in absence of complications, esp bleeding

Treatment – Nonpharmacologic
Dialysis – severe cases

Treatment – Pharmacologic [13]

Antibiotics

Amoxicillin

Ampicillin

Cephalosporins

Doxycycline

Erythromycin

Penicillin

Treatment – Surgical/Invasive

NA

Precautions

Handling specimens

Standard

Primary Prevention

Vaccine: yes

Animal immunization

Avoid contaminated water

Chemoprophylaxis for exposure

Protective clothing and footware

Rodent control

Course

Highly variable

Recovery usual

Increased mortality with advanced age and pregnancy

Notes

[1]   Severe form of leptospirosis with jaundice

[2]   Abrupt onset; often subclinical

[3]   Conjunctival suffusion is most characteristic physical feature

[4]   Esp frontal

[5]   May be severe, esp back and legs

[6]   Second phase, with meningismus

[7]   Esp trunk

[8]   Uncommon

[9]   Uncommon except in Asia

[10]   Occur in 2 phases separated by short afebrile period

[11]   50% of USA cases occur in Hawaii
[12]   Coronary arteritis and aortitis have also been found at autopsy
[13]   Uncertain efficacy

http://www.argus1.com/?lepto

Updates

_____
_____
_____
_____
_____
_____
_____
_____
_____
_____
_____
_____
_____
_____
_____

Listeriosis

Weapon
No

Alternate Names
NA

Etiology
Listeria monocytogenes

Transmission
Source: Soil, water, silage, animals, humans, food [2]
Entry: Ingestion [3]
                   Contact
Human-to-Human: Maternal – fetal
                   Fecal – oral

Predisposing/Comorbid Conditions
Advanced age
Cancer
Diabetes mellitus
Immune compromise, esp AIDS
Iron-overload states
Newborn [5]
Patients taking glucocorticoids
Pregnancy [10]
Renal disease

Demographics
Location: Gobal
Populations: All
Calendar: Year-round

Systems
Gastrointestinal
Nervous

Incubation
Invasive: 3-70 days (mean 3 weeks)
Noninvasive gastroenteritis: <1-2 days

Signs/Symptoms [1]
Abdomen – cramps
Appetite – decreased (anorexia)
Bowel movements – diarrhea
Chills
Head – pain (headache)
Mentation – fatigue
Muscles – pain (myalgia)
Nausea
Neck, post – stiff (meningismus)
Skin, hands/arms – papules [4]
Temperature, body – elevated (fever)
Vomiting

Differentiation
Includes, but not limited to:
Brain abscess
Fever of unknown origin [10]
Gastroenteritis – other causes
Meningoencephalitis – other causes

Complications
Include, but not limited to:
Acute respiratory distress syndrome (ARDS)
Brain abscess
Brain stem encephalitis (rhombencephalitis) [9]
Disseminated intravascular coagulation (DIC)
Endocarditis
Eye inflammation
Meningoencephalitis [8]
Pericarditis
Peritonitis
Pneumonia
Pregnancy-related [10]
infection of newborn [7]
miscarriage
placental rupture

> premature labor
> spontaneous abortion
> stillbirth endocarditis

Rhabdomyolysis

Sepsis

Laboratory [6] ▲

Blood culture – positive

CSF culture – positive

Stool culture – positive

ECG

NA in absence of complications

Imaging

NA in absence of complications

Other Tests

NA in absence of complications

Treatment – Nonpharmacologic

NS

Treatment – Pharmacologic

Antibiotics

> Aminoglycosides
> Ampicillin
> Penicillin
> Trimethoprim – sulfa

Treatment – Surgical/Invasive

NA in absence of complications

Precautions [6]

Standard

Primary Prevention

Vaccine: investigational

Cooking and pasteurization kill organism, but contamination can occur after cooking before packaging, so packaged cooked foods should be reheated

Pregnant women and immunocompromised patients: thorough cleaning and cooking of all foods, esp leftovers, and avoidance of soft cheeses and deli meats ▲

Course

Mortality, untreated – as high as 25% in elderly, immunocompromised, newborns ☠

Notes

[1]   Most infected persons are asymptomatic

[2]   Multiplies in refrigerated foods, esp dairy products, vegetables, meats

[3]   Contaminated food, esp soft cheese and deli meats

[4]   Direct contact with agent

[5]   Exposure to infected mother in birth canal

[6]   Laboratory personnel who are pregnant, immune deficient, or have other predisposing conditions should avoid handling specimens containing this agent ▲

[7]   Premature birth with sepsis or meningitis in term babies 2 weeks postpartum

[8]   Many atypical features common compared to other causes of meningitis, i.e., seizures, changing mental status, movement disorders

[9]   Mainly healthy adults

[10]   Esp 3rd trimester pregnancy

http://www.argus1.com/?listeria

Updates

_____
_____
_____
_____
_____
_____
_____
_____
_____
_____
_____
_____
_____
_____
_____

Lyme Disease

Weapon
No

Alternate Names
Acrodermatitis chronica atrophicans
Bannwarth syndrome
Erythema chronicum migrans
LD
Steere's disease
Tick-borne meningopolyneuritis

Etiology [1]
Borrelia burgdorferi

Transmission
Source:	*Ixodes* ticks from wild animals [14]
Entry:	Tick bite
Human-to-Human:	No

Predisposing/Comorbid Conditions
NA

Demographic
Location:	Asia, Europe, N America
Population:	All, esp children, young adults
Calendar:	Year-round, esp summer

Systems
Cardiovascular
Liver/Biliary tract/Pancreas
Lymphatic
Musculoskeletal

Nervous
Optic
Skin

Incubation
3-30 days (mean 7-10 days)

Signs/Symptoms [1]
Back, lumbar – pain
Bones – pain [8]
Breathing – diff, rest (rest dyspnea)
Chest, ant – pain, nonpleuritic rest [10]
Chills
Consciousness – loss, sudden (syncope) [9]
Cough – acute NS
Cough – nonproductive
Eyes, conjunctivae – injected
Eyes, iris – inflammed
Eyes, retina – swollen
Head, gen – pain (headache)
Heart, rate – reduced (bradycardia) [9]
Heart, rhythm – irregular [9]
Joints, local – tender [2]
Joints – pain (arthralgia) [2, 7]
Joints – swollen [2]
Liver – enlarged (hepatomegaly)
Lymph nodes – enlarged
Mentation – fatigue
Mentation – memory loss
Mentation – weakness (malaise) [3]
Mood – depression
Multiple s/s – nervous system
Muscles – pain (myalgia)
Nausea
Neck, post – pain
Neck, post – stiff
Seizures
Skin, local – macule/papule, single [4]
Skin, local – necrosis, single [4]
Skin, local – rings, red, single [4]

Skin – itching (urticaria)
Skin – red (erythema)
Spleen – enlarged
Temperature, body – elevated (fever)
Tendons – pain [8]
Testicles, bilat – enlarged
Throat – sore
Vomiting

Differentiation

Includes, but not limited to:
Acute rheumatic fever
Bell's palsy
Chronic fatigue syndrome
Multiple sclerosis
Reiter's syndrome
Rheumatoid arthritis

Complications

Include, but not limited to:
Acrodermatitis chronica atrophicans
Arthritis
Cerebellar ataxia [12]
Chorea [12]
Cranial neuritis [5, 12]
Dilated cardiomyopathy
Encephalopathy [12]
Facial palsy
Fatigue, recurrent
Keratitis
Lymphocytoma benigna cutis
Meningitis [12]
Mononeuritis multiplex [12]
Myelitis [12]
Myocarditis [6]
Pericarditis
Peripheral neuropathy [12]
Radiculopathy [12]

Laboratory

Blood IgG-specific antibodies – present
Blood IgM-specific antibodies – present

Synovial fluid protein – increased
Synovial fluid WBC – increased

Imaging
Heart – enlarged [10]

ECG
AV conduction – 1st degree block [10]
AV conduction – 2nd degree block, Mobitz I (Wenckebach) [10]
AV conduction – 3rd degree block [10]
ST-T wave – NS abnormality [10]

Other Tests
NA in absence of complications

Treatment – Nonpharmacologic
Tick removal [15] ▲

Treatment – Pharmacologic
Antibiotics [13]
      Amoxicillin
      Ceftriaxone
      Doxycycline
      Erythromycin
      Penicillin
      Tetracycline

Treatment – Surgical/Invasive
Joint fluid aspiration
Synovectomy [11]

Precautions
Standard

Primary Prevention
Vaccine: yes
Early tick removal [15] ▲
Tick-bite prevention

Course
Variable
Spontaneous resolution usual

Notes

[1]   Lyme disease is complex and highly variable in its clinical manifesta-
      tions in 3 stages: (1) localized erythema migrans; (2) involvement of
      skin, musculoskeletal, nervous, lymphatic, cardiovascular and other
      systems; and (3) chronic infection

[2]   Esp knees and other large joints; frank arthritis often occurs if no
      antibiotic treatment given initially

[3]   May be severe

[4]   Erythema chronicum migrans; esp thigh, groin, axilla; usually warm
      but not painful; may secondarily expand into multiple lesions

[5]   Esp bilateral facial palsy

[6]   Includes varying degrees of heart block

[7]   Migratory early in course; frank arthritis later

[8]   Migratory

[9]   Due to varying degress of heart block with cardiac involvement

[10] Due to myocarditis; usually short-lived

[11] Only long-term unresolving joint effusions

[12] Neurological complications

[13] Variable depending on specific involvement and severity

[14] *Ioxides* also transmits *Babesia microtic* (babesiosis) and *Anaplasma
      phagocytophilium* (ehrlichiosis) which can cause coinfection with
      Lyme disease

[15] Within 24 hours after attachment can be preventative ▲

http://www.argus1.com/?lyme

Updates

_____
_____
_____
_____
_____
_____
_____
_____
_____
_____
_____
_____

Lymphocytic Choriomeningitis

Weapon
CDC Bioterrorism Category: A

Alternate Names
LCM
Lymphocytic meningitis

Etiology
Lymphocytic choriomeningitis virus (arenavirus)

Viremia infects multiple organ systems with predilection for central nervous system, followed by inflammatory response

Transmission
Source:	Aerosolized rodent (mouse, hamster) waste or saliva
Entry:	Ingestion of contaminated food
	Direct exposure of open skin lesions to infected blood
	Fetal circulation
Human-to-Human:	Mother-fetus; organ transplant

Predisposing/Comorbid Conditions
Skin abrasion

Demographics
Location:	Global, esp Europe, Americas, Japan, Australia
Populations:	All
Calendar:	Year-round, usually autumn

Systems
Musculoskeletal
Nervous
Skin

Incubation
1-3 weeks

Signs/Symptoms [1]
Appetite – decreased (anorexia)
Back, lumbar – pain
Chest, ant – pain, nonpleuritic rest
Chills
Cough – nonproductive
Mentation – lightheaded
Extremities, sensations – abnormal (dysesthesias) [2]
Eyes, light sensitivity – increased (photophobia)
Eyes, retroorbital – pain
Face, parotid – pain [2]
Hair, head – loss (alopecia) [2]
Head – pain (headache)
Heart rate – decreased relative to fever (relative bradycardia)
Joints, hand – pain [2]
Joints, hand – swollen [2, 3]
Joints – pain (arthralgia)
Lymph nodes – enlarged
Mentation – confusion [2]
Mentation – weakness (malaise)
Muscles – pain (myalgia)
Muscles – paralysis [2, 4]
Nausea
Neck, post – stiff (meningismus) [2]
Skin – rash, macular/papular [2]
Skin – rash, red (erythematous) [2]
Temperature, body – elevated (fever)
Testicles, bilat – pain [2]
Throat – injected
Throat – sore
Vomiting

Differentiation
Includes, but not limited to:
Other forms of encephalitis
Other forms of meningitis
Other viral hemorrhagic fevers

Complications

Include, but not limited to:
  Acute hydrocephalus
  Alopecia
  Arthritis
  Encephalomyelitis
  Myelitis
  Myocarditis
  Nerve deafness
  Orchitis
  Pregnancy:
      Abortion
      Congenital chorioretinitis
      Congenital hydrocephalus
      Mental retardation

Laboratory [6] ▲

  Blood ELISA antibodies – positive
  Blood liver enzymes – increased
  Blood platelets, total – decreased (thrombocytopenia)
  Blood WBC, total – decreased (leukopenia)
  CSF ELISA antibody titer – positive
  CSF glucose – decreased
  CSF lymphocytes – increased
  CSF protein – increased

ECG

  NA in absence of complications, esp myocarditis

Imaging

  NA in absence of complications

Other Tests

  NA in absence of complications

Treatment – Nonpharmacologic

  NS

Treatment – Pharmacologic

  Ribavirin [5]

Treatment – Surgical/Invasive

NA in absence of complications

Precautions

BSL-4 laboratory procedures ▲
Standard

Primary Prevention

Vaccine: no
Rodent control and handling of rodents

Course

Mortality <1%

Notes

[1]   Course occurs in two phases, first phase lasting up to 1 week, with 1-2 day interlude, followed by second phase with neurological features
[2]   Phase 2
[3]   MIP and PIP joints
[4]   Rare
[5]   Consider for severe infection
[6]   BSL-3 procedures

http://www.argus1.com/?lympchor

Updates

_____
_____
_____
_____
_____
_____
_____
_____
_____
_____
_____
_____
_____
_____

Malaria

Weapon
No

Alternate Names
Ague
Marsh fever

Etiology
P falciparum
P malariae
P ovale
P vivax

Transmission
Source:	Humans
Entry:	Mosquito bite [5]
	Blood transfusion
Human-to Human:	Via mosquito only

Predisposing/Comorbid Conditions
HIV

Demographics
Location:	Tropics and subtropics
Populations:	All, esp children; pregnant women risk complications
Calendar:	Year-round, esp after rain in dry areas

Systems
Hematopoietic/immune
Liver/Biliary tract/Pancreas
Nervous

Incubation [3]

P falciparum:	7-14 days
P malariae:	7-30 days
P ovale:	8-14 days
P vivax:	8-14 days

Signs/Symptoms [6, 8]

Abdomen – pain
Abdomen – tender
Appetite – decreased (anorexia)
Arterial pressure, diastolic – decreased
Arterial pressure, systolic – decreased
Back, gen – pain
Bowel movements – blood or black (hematochezia) (melena)
Bowel movements – diarrhea
Chills
Consciousness – altered
Cough – nonproductive
Eyes, retina – hemorrhage
Head – pain (headache)
Heart rate – increased (tachycardia)
Joints – pain (arthralgia)
Liver – enlarged (hepatomegaly)
Lymph nodes – enlarged
Mentation – confusion
Mentation – delirium
Mentation – fatigue
Mentation – sleepy (somnolence)
Mentation – weakness (malaise)
Muscles – pain (myalgia)
Nausea
Seizures
Skin color – pallor
Skin color – yellow (jaundice)
Sleep – disturbed (insomnia)
Spleen – enlarged (splenomegaly)
Sweating – increased (hyperhydrosis)
Temperature, body – elevated (fever)
Vomiting

Differentiation

Includes, but not limited to:
Other recurrent febrile illnesses

Complications

Include, but not limited to:
Anemia
Blackwater fever [1]
Cerebral malaria
Cognitive impairment
Gastroenteritis
Hypoglycemia
Liver failure
Metabolic acidosis
Noncardiac pulmonary edema
Pregnancy:
      fetal death ☠
      maternal death ☠
      miscarriage
      neonatal death ☠
Renal failure
Respiratory distress
Shock
Spleen rupture

Laboratory

Blood bilirubin – increased
Blood creatinine – increased
Blood glucose – decreased (hypoglycemia)
Blood Hgb/Hct – decreased (anemia)
Blood liver enzymes – increased
Blood lymphocytes – decreased (lymphopenia) [2]
Blood pH – decreased (metabolic acidosis)
Blood platelets – decreased (thrombocytopenia)
Blood sodium – decreased (hyponatremia)
Blood WBC – decreased (leukopenia)
Blood WBC – increased (leukocytosis)
Urine hemoglobin – present (hemoglobinuria)
Urine protein – present (proteinuria)

ECG
Rate – rapid (sinus tachycardia)

Imaging
NS in absence of complications

Other Tests
Demonstration of parasite in bloodstream (Giemsa stain)
Rapid dipstick test for *plasmodium* protein or LDH

Treatment – Nonpharmacologic
NS

Treatment – Pharmacologic [8, 9] ▲
Artemether
Atovaquone
Chloroquine
Doxycycline
Lumefantine
Primaquine
Proguanil
Quinidine
Quinine

Treatment – Surgical/Invasive
NA in absense of complications

Precautions
Needle disposal ▲

Primary Prevention
Vaccine: no
Chemoprophylaxis [9]
Mosquito control and exposure
Physical barriers to mosquito bites [4] ▲
Pregnant women should exercise maximum protection, including
    avoiding malarious areas whenever possible ▲

Course
Variable

Notes

[1]   Characterized by intravascular hemolysis and hemoglobinuria

[2]   Total WBC may be normal

[3]   Shorter with transmission by transfusion and longer with *p vivax* in temperate climates; onset delayed with partial chemoprophylaxis

[4]   Includes not going out at night, wearing light-colored clothes covering all skin, using repellants

[5]   Female *anopheles* mosquito

[6]   May be cyclical

[7]   Body loss due to inappropriate ADH secretion

[8]   Begin treatment as soon as diagnosis suspected ▲

[9]   Consult current guidelines as multiple drug regimens are used and recommendations often change ▲

http://www.argus1.com/?malaria

Updates

_____

_____

_____

_____

_____

_____

_____

_____

_____

_____

_____

_____

_____

Marburg Hemorrhagic Fever

Weapon
CDC Bioterrorism Category: A

Alternate Names
African hemorrhagic fever

Etiology
Marburg filovirus (*Filoviridae* virus)

Initially infects lymphatic system, with dissemination to testes, ovaries, and liver, with secondary, severe effects on blood coagulation

Transmission
Source: Monkeys, bats

Entry: Contact with animals or materials contaminated with infectious blood or body secretions

Human-to-Human: Yes

Predisposing/Comorbid Conditions
NA

Demographics
Location: Africa, esp Congo

Populations: Monkey handlers, laboratory personnel, caregivers

Calendar: Year-round

Systems
Coagulation

Liver/Biliary tract/Pancreas

Renal/Genitourinary

Incubation
5-10 days

Signs/Symptoms [7]
Abdomen – pain
Appetite – reduced (anorexia)
Bowel movements, stool – blood or black (hematochezia) (melena)
Bowel movements – diarrhea
Breathing – rapid (tachypnea)
Chills
Eyes, conjunctivae – injected
Eyes – burning, itching
Fatigue
Head – pain (headache)
Hiccups [1]
Joints – pain (arthralgia)
Mentation – apathetic
Mentation – confused
Mentation – weakness (malaise)
Mouth, gingiva – bleeding
Mouth, mucosa – hemorrhage
Mouth, mucosa – ulcers
Muscles – pain (myalgia)
Nausea
Nose – blood (epistaxis)
Skin – petechiae
Skin – rash, desquamating
Skin – rash, macular/papular [3]
Sputum – blood (hemoptysis)
Swallowing – difficult (dysphagia)
Swallowing – pain (odynophagia)
Temperature, body – elevated (fever)
Throat – sore
Vagina – blood
Vomiting
Vomiting – blood (hematemesis)
Weight – loss

Differentiation
Includes, but not limited to:
Ebola and other viral hemorrhagic fevers

Malaria
Rickettsial diseases
Typhoid fever

Complications

Include, but not limited to:
Blindness
Disseminated intravascular coagulation (DIC)
Hepatitis, recurrent
Liver failure
Massive hemorrhage
Multi-organ failure
Myocarditis
Orchitis
Pancreatitis
Parotitis
Renal failure
Shock
Spontaneous abortion
Transverse myelitis
Uveitis

Laboratory [6] ▲

Blood amylase – increased
Blood creatinine – increased
Blood ELISA IgG antibodies – positive (2nd week)
Blood liver enzymes – increased
Blood lymphocytes – decreased (lymphopenia)
Blood platelets, total – decreased (thrombocytopenia)
Blood prothrombin time – increased
Blood WBC – decreased (leukopenia)
Blood WBC – left shift [4]
Urine protein – present (proteinuria)

ECG

NS [5]

Imaging

NA in absence of complications

Other Tests

NA in absence of complications

Treatment – Nonpharmacologic
NS

Treatment – Pharmacologic
NS
Replace blood or clotting factors

Treatment – Surgical/Invasive
NA

Precautions
BSL-4 procedures ▲

Primary Prevention
Vaccine: no

Course
About 25% fatal [2] ☠

Notes
[1]   Esp fatal cases ☠
[2]   May have been higher in outbreak in Angola
[3]   Esp trunk, back
[4]   Early in course
[5]   May be abnormal if myocarditis present
[6]   BSL-4 procedures ▲
[7]   Sudden onset

http://www.argus1.com/?marburg

Updates

Melioidosis

Weapon
CDC Bioterrorism Category: B

Alternate Names
Pseudoglanders
Whitmore's disease

Etiology
Burkholder pseudomallei

Initial local infection in skin or lungs with intracellular multiplication; may become disseminated via bloodstream, with septic shock

Transmission
Source: Soil
Entry: Contact through skin wound
                     Inhalation
                     Ingestion
Human-to-Human: Yes

Predisposing/Comorbid Conditions
Chronic conditions, i.e., HIV, renal failure, diabetes mellitus, chronic lung disease, alcohol excess

Demographics
Location: Global, esp SE Asia, Northern Australia, S Pacific, China, Africa, India, Middle East
Populations: All, esp debilitated; military serving in endemic areas
Calendar: Year-round

Systems
Musculoskeletal
Renal/Genitourinary
Respiratory – lower
Skin

Time to Clinical Onset

Days – years

Signs/Symptoms (Acute form) [1]

Appetite – decreased (anorexia)
Breath sounds – coarse (rhonchi)
Breath sounds – crackling (rales)
Breathing – diff, rest (rest dyspnea)
Chest, gen – pain, pleuritic
Chills
Cough – productive
Head – pain (headache)
Lymph nodes, regional – enlarged
Mentation – confused
Mentation – weakness (malaise)
Muscles – pain (myalgia)
Muscles – tender
Skin – nodule
Skin – ulcer, single
Skin – rash, papular
Skin – rash, pruritic
Skin – rash, pustular
Sputum – blood (hemoptysis)
Sputum – purulent
Temperature, body – elevated (fever)

Differentiation (Acute form)

Includes, but not limited to:
Glanders
Other causes of pulmonary infection
Tuberculosis

Complications

Include, but not limited to:
Chronic suppurative infection involving many organs, i.e., brain,
bone, joints, liver, parotid, spleen
Septicemia

Laboratory [2]

Blood culture – positive

Blood IgM-specific antibodies – present
Blood lymphocytes – increased (lymphocytosis)
Blood serology – positive
Blood WBC – increased (leukocytosis)
Skin culture – positive
Skin stain – positive
Sputum culture – positive
Sputum stain – positive
Urine culture – positive

ECG
NA in absence of complications

Imaging
Chest x-ray
        cavitation
        infiltrates – apical
        nodules – diffuse, miliary

Other Tests
NA in absence of complications

Treatment – Nonpharmacologic
NS

Treatment – Pharmacologic
Antibiotics
        Ceftazadime
        Doxycycline
        Imipenem
        Meropenem
        Trimethoprim – sulfa

Treatment – Surgical/Invasive
NA in absence of complications

Precautions
Contact
Standard

Primary Prevention

Vaccine: no

Barrier techniques with soil contact [3]

Course

Recovery usual; death may occur secondary to septicimea ☠

Notes

[1] Melioidosis may present in an acute form (described) with skin or pulmonary manifestations or multi-organ absesses anywhere in the body; or in a chronic form with protean manifestations

[2] Definitive diagnosis requires positive culture of infected site

[3] Shoes, gloves

[4] May be severe

http://www.argus1.com/?melioidosis

Updates

_____
_____
_____
_____
_____
_____
_____
_____
_____
_____
_____
_____
_____
_____
_____
_____
_____
_____
_____
_____

Meningococcemia

Weapon
No

Alternate Names
Purpura fulminans [1]
Waterhouse-Friderichsen syndrome [1]

Etiology
Neisseria meningitidis

Transmission
Source:	Secretions from infected humans
Entry:	Mucosal contact
Human-to-Human:	Yes

Predisposing/Comorbid Conditions
Asplenia
Enteropathy
Genetic complement C5-C9 deficiency
Hepatic disease
HIV
Immunoglobulin deficiency
Multiple myeloma
Nephrotic syndrome
Systemic lupus erythematosis

Demographics
Location:	Global, esp sub-Saharan Africa [12]
Populations:	All – esp infants, late teens-early 20's, bacteriologists, military recruits, residents of college dormitories [13]
Calendar:	Year-round, peak late winter – early spring

Systems

Hematopoietic/Immune
Nervous
Skin

Incubation

2-10 days

Signs/Symptoms [2]

Appetite – decreased (anorexia)
Arterial press – low (hypotension)
Chills
Consciousness – loss, prolonged (coma)
Cough – acute NS [3]
Eyes, light sensitivity – increased (photophobia)
Head – pain (headache)
Heart rate – increased (tachycardia)
Joints – pain (arthralgia)
Mentation – delirium [1]
Mentation – sleepy (somnolence)
Mentation – weak (malaise)
Mood – restless/irritable [1]
Muscles – pain (myalgia)
Nausea
Neck, post – stiff (meningismus)
Skin, gen – rash, ecchymotic [1, 6]
Skin – rash, macular/papular
Skin – rash, petechiae [4]
Skin – rash, purpura [1, 6]
Skin – rash, pustular [1]
Skin – rash, urticarial[7]
Temperature, body – elevated (fever) [5]
Temperature, body – low [5]
Throat – injected
Throat – sore [3]
Vomiting

Differentiation

Includes, but not limited to:
Dengue fever
Infective endocarditis

Other causes of meningitis
Rocky Mountain spotted fever
Thrombotic thrombocytopenic purpura

Complications

Include, but not limited to:

Adrenal failure [1]
Arthritis – immune complex
Arthritis – septic
Congestive heart failure
Conjunctivitis
Deafness
Disseminated intravascular coagulation (DIC)
Endocarditis
Endometritis
Epiglottitis
Hepatic failure
Herpes labialis
Limb gangrene
Meningitis
Myocarditis
Osteomyelitis
Pericarditis
Renal failure
Respiratory failure
Seizures
Sinusitis
Thrombocytopenia
Urethritis
Vascular collapse
Vascular thrombosis

Laboratory [15] ▲

Blood culture – positive [8]
Blood latex agglutination – positive [1]
Blood platelets– decreased (thrombocytopenia) [1]
Blood WBC – increased (leukocytosis)
Blood WBC – left shift
CSF bacterial stain – positive [9]
CSF culture – positive [9]
CSF glucose – decreased [9]

CSF latex agglutination – positive [10]
CSF protein – increased [9]
CSF WBC – increased [9]
Skin culture – positive

ECG
NA in absence of complications

Imaging
NA in absence of complications

Other Tests
NA in absence of complications

Treatment – Nonpharmacologic
Cardiac support
Fluids and electrolytes
Ventilation

Treatment – Pharmacologic
Antibiotics [16] ▲
      Cephalosporins – third generation
      Chloramphenicol
      Penicillin G
Corticosteroids (?) [13]
Platelets and clotting factors

Treatment – Surgical/Invasive
NA in absence of complications

Precautions
Standard [15] ▲

Primary Prevention
Vaccine: yes
      college students
      travelers
      pregnant women
Chemoprophylaxis [16] ▲
Living space ventilation
Reduce/eliminate crowded living conditions
Reduce/eliminate secretion exposure from infected persons

Course

Mortality 5-10% [14] ☠

Notes

[1]   Waterhouse-Friderichsen (WF) or pupura fulminans severe toxic extension of meningococcemia, in about 10% of cases

[2]   Initial clinical appearance may be mild, resembling a viral URI

[3]   Upper respiratory s/s often precede septicemia

[4]   Usually in crops on ankles, wrists, axillae, flanks, then extending to other areas, sparing palms and soles

[5]   Moderate except high in WF; normal or low temperature indicates poor prognosis

[6]   Esp pressure points, with necrotic centers

[7]   Initial cutaneous lesions

[8]   75%

[9]   With leptomeningeal involvement

[10]   For capsular polysaccharide

[11]   "Meningitis belt" with cyclic, major epidemics

[12]   Affects all ages in epidemics

[13]   Efficacy uncertain

[14]   Up to 90% with DIC

[15]   Caution in handling specimens ▲

[16]   Consult current guidelines before prescribing ▲

http://www.argus1.com/?menin

Updates

_____
_____
_____
_____
_____
_____
_____
_____
_____
_____
_____
_____

Monkeypox

Weapon
No

Alternate Names
NA

Etiology
Monkeypox virus, an orthopoxvirus

Transmission

Source:	Primates, rodents, rabbits, humans [4]
Entry:	Animal bite
	Contact with secretions from infected animal
	Inhalation
Human-to-Human:	Yes [5]

Predisposing/Comorbid Conditions
NA

Demographics

Locations:	Most cases reported in Central Africa; 1 outbreak in USA midwest [6]
Populations:	All
Calendar:	Year-round

Systems
Lymphatic
Skin

Incubation
7-20 days

Signs/Symptoms

Back – pain
Breathing – diff, rest (rest dyspnea)
Chills
Cough – nonproductive
Hair, head – loss (alopecia) [1]
Head – pain (headache)
Lymph nodes – enlarged [7]
Mentation – fatigue
Muscles – pain (myalgia)
Nausea
Skin, sweating – increased (hyperhidrosis)
Skin – rash, crusting [2, 3]
Skin – rash, papular [2, 3]
Skin – rash, pustular [2, 3]
Skin – rash, vesicular [2, 3]
Skin – ulcers [2]
Temperature, body – elevated (fever)
Throat – sore
Vomiting

Differentiation

Includes, but not limited to:

Chickenpox
Cowpox
Smallpox
Vaccinia

Complications

Bacterial skin infection
Encephalitis
Keratitis
Pulmonary

Laboratory [9] ▲

NS in absence of complications

ECG

NA in absence of complications

Imaging
NA in absence of complications

Other Tests
NA in absence of complications

Treatment – Nonpharmacologic
NS

Treatment – Pharmacologic
NS

Treatment – Surgical/Invasive
NA

Precautions
BSL-2 or BSL-3 procedures ▲
Standard

Primary Prevention
Vaccine: no [8]
Avoid contact with suspect animals ▲
Handwashing after contact with suspect animal ▲
Infection control

Course
Duration – 2-4 weeks
Mortality in Africa – up to 10% ☠

Notes
[1]   May occur in acute stage illness
[2]   Multiple stages may exist concurrently
[3]   Head, trunk, extremities; may begin on soles or generalized
[4]   Monkeys in Africa; prairie dogs in USA; all animals may be suspect
[5]   Respiratory droplets; body fluids; direct contact
[6]   In 2003 from infected prairie dogs in Wisconsin, Illinois, Indiana
[7]   Differentiating point from smallpox, which does not cause lymphadenopathy
[8]   Smallpox vaccination may convey some preventative effect if given soon after exposure
[9]   BSL-2 or BSL-3 procedures ▲

http://www.argus1.com/?monkey

Updates

_____
_____
_____
_____
_____
_____
_____
_____
_____
_____
_____
_____
_____
_____
_____
_____
_____
_____
_____
_____
_____
_____
_____

Mumps

Weapon
No

Alternate Names
Epidemic parotitis
Infectious parotitis

Etiology
Mumps virus (genus paramyxovirus)

Transmission
Source: Humans
Entry: Direct contact with infected saliva
Human-to-Human: Yes

Predisposing/Comorbid Conditions
NA

Demographic
Location: Global
Population: All persons unvaccinated/without prior infection
Calendar: Year-round, peak winter and spring

Systems
Nervous
Genitourinary
Oropharynx

Incubation
14-21 days

Signs/Symptoms

Appetite – decreased (anorexia) [3]
Cough – nonproductive [4]
Ears – pain
Face, jaw – tender [1, 2]
Face, parotid glands – enlarged [1]
Face, parotid glands – pain [1, 5]
Face, parotid glands – tender
Neck, submandibular glands – pain
Neck, submandibular glands – enlarged
Neck, submandibular glands – tender
Head – pain (headache) [3]
Mentation – weak (malaise)
Mouth, chewing – pain [5]
Mouth, Stensen's duct – inflammation
Muscles – pain (myalgia) [3]
Swallowing – pain (odynophagia) [5]
Temperature, body – elevated (fever) [3]

Differentiation

Includes, but not limited to:

Other infectious causes of parotid swelling [8]
Noninfectious causes of parotid swelling [9]

Complications

Include, but not limited to:

Arthritis
Deafness
Encephalitis
Fetal death – 1st trimester
Mastitis
Meningitis – aseptic
Myocarditis
Nephritis
Oophoritis
Orchitis
Pancreatitis

Laboratory

Blood amylase – increased

Blood IgG-specific antibodies – present
Blood IgM-specific antibodies – present [6]

ECG [7]
NS ST-T wave changes
Prolonged PR interval

Imaging
NA in absence of complications

Other Tests
NA in absence of complications

Treatment – Nonpharmacologic
Parotid warm/cold packs
Soft diet

Treatment – Pharmacologic
NS

Treatment – Surgical/Invasive
NA in absence of complications

Precautions
Standard

Primary Prevention
Vaccine: yes
Avoid exposure to high risk persons such as those with AIDS,
pregnancy ▲

Course
Complete recovery usual

Notes
[1]   Unilateral or bilateral
[2]   Angle of jaw
[3]   Prodromal symptom

[4] May present as lower respiratory illness, esp preschool children

[5] Esp with acidic drinks

[6] Positive in first few days, peak 1 week

[7] May be abnormal in mumps myocarditis, which occurs in up to 15% of cases

[8] Coxsackie, influenza, parainfluenza, HIV, staphylococcus

[9] Drugs, diabetes, uremia, malnutrition, cirrhosis

http://www.argus1.com/?mumps

Updates

_____
_____
_____
_____
_____
_____
_____
_____
_____
_____
_____
_____
_____
_____
_____
_____
_____
_____
_____

OMSK Hemorrhagic Fever

Weapon
CDC Bioterrorism Category: A

Alternate Names
OHF

Etiology
OMSK hemorrhagic fever virus (a flaviviridae virus)

Causes small blood vessel thrombi, RBC extravasation, surrounding tissue edema

Transmission
Source:	Ticks, muskrats, rodents
Entry:	Tick bite
	Direct contact
	Ingestion of contaminated water
Human-to-Human:	No

Predisposing/Comorbid Conditions
NA

Demographic
Location:	Western Siberia
Population:	All, esp muskrat trappers
Calendar:	Peak in late spring and late summer

Systems
Coagulation
Nervous

Incubation
3-8 days

Signs/Symptoms
Bowel movements, stool – blood or black (hematochezia) (melena)

Chills

Extremities, lower – pain

Extremities, upper – pain

Eyes, conjunctivae – blood

Head – pain (headache)

Lymph nodes, anterior cervical – enlarged

Mentation – confusion

Mentation – delirium

Mentation – weakness (malaise)

Mouth, soft palate – erruption, papulovesicular

Muscles – pain (myalgia)

Muscles – tremors, intention

Neck, posterior – stiff (meningismus)

Nose – blood (epistaxis)

Sputum – blood (hemoptysis)

Temperature, body – elevated (fever)

Urine – blood (hematuria)

Vagina – blood

Vomiting – blood (hematemesis)

Differentiation
Includes, but not limited to:

Coagulopathies

Encephalitis

Other viral hemorrhagic fevers

Complications
Include, but not limited to:

Alopecia

Hearing loss

Neuropsychiatric changes

Pneumonia

Shock

Laboratory [1] ▲
Blood culture – positive
Blood IgM specific antibodies – positive
Blood platelets – decreased (thrombocytopenia) [2]
Blood WBC – decreased (leukopenia) [2]
Urine blood – positive
Urine protein – present (proteinuria)

ECG
NA in absence of complications

Imaging
NA in absence of complications

Other Tests
NA in absence of complications

Treatment – Nonpharmacologic
Fluids, electrolytes

Treatment – Pharmacologic
NS

Treatment – Surgical/Invasive
NA

Precautions
BSL-4 procedures ▲
Standard

Primary Prevention
Vaccine: experimental
Tick bite prevention

Course
<5% mortality

Notes

[1]   BSL-4 procedures ▲

[2]   Decrease may be marked

http://www.argus1.com/?omsk

Updates

_____

_____

_____

_____

_____

_____

_____

_____

_____

_____

_____

_____

_____

_____

_____

_____

_____

_____

_____

_____

Parvovirus B19

Weapon
No

Alternate Names
Academy rash
Erythema infectiosum
Fifth disease
Slapped cheek disease
Sticker's disease

Etiology
Human parvovirus B19

Transmission
Source:	Humans
Entry:	Inhalation
	Maternal-fetal
	Transfusion
Human-to-Human:	Yes [10]

Predisposing/Comorbid Conditions [12]
Congenital hemolytic anemia
Immune deficiency
Pregnancy

Demographics
Location:	Global
Populations:	All, esp children
Calendar:	Late winter-early spring in epidemics

Systems
Hematopoietic
Musculoskeletal
Skin

Incubation

4-20 days

Signs/Symptoms [9]

Appetite – decreased (anorexia) [1]
Bowel movements – diarrhea [1]
Cough – nonproductive [1]
Head – pain (headache) [1]
Joints – pain (arthralgia) [2]
Joints – swelling [2]
Mentation – weak (malaise) [1]
Mouth, mucosa – ulcers [3]
Muscles – pain (myalgia)
Muscles – stiffness
Nausea [1]
Nose, drainage – increased (rhinorrhea, coryza) [1]
Nose – congested [1]
Skin, face – rash, red (erythema) [4]
Skin – rash, macular/papular [5]
Skin – rash, petechiae [6]
Skin – rash, pruritic [13]
Skin – rash, purpura [6]
Skin – rash, red (erythematous) [5]
Skin – rash, vesicular [6]
Temperature, body – elevated (fever) [1]

Differentiation

Includes, but not limited to:

Other causes of arthritis [11]
Other causes of hemorrhagic/vesicular/maculopapular rashes
Scarlet fever

Complications

Include, but not limited to:

Aplastic crisis [7]
Chronic infection [8]
Encephalitis
Hypdrops fetalis
Spontaneous abortion

Laboratory
Blood IgG-specific antibodies – positive
Blood IgM-specific antibodies – positive
Blood WBC – increased (leukocytosis)
Bone marrow – amorphic pronormoblast inclusions

ECG
NA in absence of complications

Imaging
NA in absence of complications

Other Tests
NA in absence of complications

Treatment – Nonpharmacologic
NS

Treatment – Pharmacologic
NS

Treatment – Surgical/Invasive
NA

Precautions
Aerosol barriers before rash appears
Standard

Primary Prevention
Vaccine: in development

Course
Spontaneous resolution in days-weeks, although rash or arthritis can recur or persist longer

Notes
[1]   Prodromal phase
[2]   Joint symptoms usually last 2-3 weeks, but sometimes can persist for several months

[3]   May resemble Koplik's spots of measles

[4]   "Slapped face" with sharp, raised borders sparing circumoral area and bridge of nose; appears between prodromal phase and before onset of rash on body

[5]   Esp trunk, buttocks, extremities; has lacy, reticular pattern; may recur with cold, sunlight, bathing, exercise, stress

[6]   May occur in some cases

[7]   Persons with congenital hemolytic anemias

[8]   Immunocompromised persons, including HIV and transplant recipients

[9]   Most infected persons are asymptomatic

[10] Occurs only in prodromal phase (prior to onset of rash)

[11] Esp juvenile rheumatoid arthritis

[12] Increased risk of complications

[13] Esp hands and feet

www.argus1.com/?parvo

Updates

_____

_____

_____

_____

_____

_____

_____

_____

_____

_____

_____

_____

_____

_____

_____

_____

_____

_____

_____

Plague

Weapon
CDC Bioterrorism Category: A

Alternate Names
Black death

Etiology
Yersinia pestis [10]

Inhaled or multipy in lymph nodes draining bite site leading to lymph node destruction (bubo), septicemia and toxemia; septicemia can cause secondary pneumonic, pharyngitic, and meningitic forms

Transmission
Source:	Rodents
Entry:	Flea bites or directly by bites of rats, other rodents, and cats
	Inhalation
Human-to-Human:	Yes

Predisposing/Comorbid Conditions
NA

Demographic
Location:	Global except Australia [7]
Populations:	Crowded living conditions, cold temperatures, high humidity
Calendar:	Year-round, esp warm seasons

Systems
Lymphatic
Nervous
Respiratory – lower

Incubation
1-6 days

Signs/Symptoms [5]
Abdomen – pain
Bowel movements – diarrhea
Breath sounds – coarse (rhonchi) [p]
Breath sounds – crackles (rales) [p]
Breathing – diff, rest (rest dyspnea) [p]
Breathing – rapid (tachypnea) [p]
Chest – pain, pleuritic [p]
Chills
Cough – productive
Digits – gangrenous [1] [s]
Head – pain (headache)
Heart rate – increased (tachycardia)
Liver – large (hepatomegaly)
Lymph nodes, ant cervical – enlarged [t]
Lymph nodes, regional – break down (suppurate) [b]
Lymph nodes, regional – enlarged [2] [b]
Lymph nodes, regional – tender [2] [b]
Lymph nodes, regional – skin overlying red/hot [2] [b]
Mentation – confusion
Mentation – delirium
Mentation – weak (malaise)
Mood – restless/irritable
Muscles, movement – incoordinated (ataxia)
Muscles – pain (myalgia)
Muscles – weak
Nausea
Neck, post – stiff (meningismus)
Nose – gangrene [1] [s]
Seizures
Skin – rash, purpura [s]
Sleep – disturbed (insomnia)
Speech – disturbed (dysphasia)
Spleen – large (splenomegaly)
Sputum – blood (hemoptysis) [p]
Sputum – clear [p]

Sputum – purulent [p]
Temperature, body – elevated (fever)
Throat – sore [t]
Vomiting [p]

Differentiation
Includes, but not limited to:
Acute abdomen
Other causes of lymphadenitis
Other causes of pneumonia
Other causes of meningitis

Complications
Include, but not limited to:
Cellulitis
Coma
Disseminated intravascular coagulation (DIC)
Meningitis
Shock – septic [11]
Skin abscess

Laboratory [8] ▲
Blood bacterial stain – positive
Blood bilirubin – increased
Blood coagulation – abnormal
Blood culture – positive
Blood glucose – decreased
Blood IgG-specific antibodies – present
Blood liver enzymes – increased
Blood specific antigen – positive
Blood WBC – increased (leukocytosis)
Lymph node culture – positive (b)
Sputum culture – positive (p)
Sputum stain – positive (p)

ECG
NA in absence of complications

Imaging
Lungs, parenchyma – consolidation (p)
Lungs, parenchyma – infiltrates (p)

Other Tests
NA in absence of complications

Treatment – Nonpharmacologic
Fluids and electrolytes
Ventilation

Treatment – Pharmacologic
Antibiotics [4]
    Chloramphenicol [3]
    Doxycycline
    Fluroquinolones
    Gentamicin
    Streptomycin
    Sulfonamides

Treatment – Surgical/Invasive
NA in absence of complications

Precautions
Isolation of patient and contacts ▲
Droplet precautions [9]
Standard

Primary Prevention [8]
Vaccine: yes
Animal reservoir control
Environmental control
Post exposure antibiotic prophylaxis
Avoid travel to endemic/epidemic areas or take appropriate precautions when doing so

Course
Treated mortality – 15% ☠
Untreated mortality – 50-90% ☠

Notes
[b]   Bubonic form
[p]   Pneumonic form
[t]   Pharyngitic form

[s]   Septicemic form
[1]   Hence "black death"
[2]   The bubo: most common in groin, axilla, neck
[3]   Esp meningitis
[4]   Consult current guidelines as protocols may vary according to form of infection; relative efficacies of agents are uncertain
[5]   All forms
[6]   Wright, Giemsa, Wayne bipolar staining
[7]   Most recent outbreaks in Asia
[8]   Level BSL-3 lab procedures ▲
[9]   Includes breathing masks for 48 hours after treatment begun
[10]   Gram-negative bacillus
[11]   May occur without bubo – termed "primary septicemic plague"

http://www.argus1.com/?plague

Updates

Psittacosis

Weapon
CDC Bioterrorism Category: B

Alternate Names
Avian chlamydiosis
Ornithosis
Parrot fever

Etiology
Chlamydia psittaci

Transmission
Source: Birds, esp parrots, parakeets, love birds, turkeys
Entry: Inhalation
Human-to-Human: Rare

Predisposing/Comorbid Conditions
NA

Demographics
Location: Global
Populations: All, esp bird owners and handlers
Calendar: Year-round

Systems
Respiratory – lower
Respiratory – upper

Incubation
1-4 weeks

Signs/Symptoms

Abdomen – distention [1]

Abdomen – pain

Appetite – decreased (anorexia)

Back – stiffness

Bowel movements – constipation

Bowel movements – diarrhea [1]

Breathing – difficult (dyspnea)

Breathing – rapid (tachypnea)

Chest – friction rub

Chest – pain, pleuritic

Chest – rales

Chills

Consciousness – loss, prolonged (coma) [2]

Cough – nonproductive

Cough – productive [1]

Ears, hearing – decreased

Ears – ringing (tinnitus)

Eyes, vision – light sensitivity, increased (photophobia)

Head – pain (headache) [3]

Heart rate – slow relative to fever (relative bradycardia)

Joints – pain (arthralgia)

Liver – enlarged (hepatomegaly) [4]

Lymph nodes, anterior cervical – enlarged

Mentation – confusion

Mentation – delirium

Mentation – feeling of weakness (malaise)

Mood – depressed

Mood – lethargic, slowed

Mood – restless, irritable

Mouth, palate – petechiae

Muscles, back – spasm

Muscles – pain (myalgia)

Muscles – tender

Nausea

Neck, posterior – stiff (meningismus)

Nose – blood (epistaxis)

Skin color – yellow (jaundice) [4]

Skin – rash, macular [5]

Sleep – disturbed (insomnia)

Spleen – enlarged (splenomegaly)
Sputum – blood (hemoptysis) [1]
Sweating – increased (hyperhydrosis)
Temperature, body – elevated (fever)
Throat – injected
Throat – sore
Vomiting

Differentiation

Includes, but not limited to:
Chlamydia pneumoniae
Coxiella burnetti
Infectious mononucleosis
Influenza
Legionnaires' disease
Meningitis
Mycoplasma pneumonia
Q fever
Tularemia
Typhoid fever
Viral pneumonias

Complications

Include, but not limited to:
Acute respiratory distress syndrome (ARDS)
Anemia, hemolytic
Arthritis
Dilated cardiomyopathy
Disseminated intravascular coagulation (DIC)
Encephalitis
Endocarditis
Glomerulonephritis
Hepatitis
Keratoconjunctivitis
Myocarditis
Pancreatitis
Pericarditis
Pregnancy – related [8]
Pulmonary infarction
Thrombophlebitis

Thyroiditis
Transverse myelitis

Laboratory [7] ▲

Blood alkaline phosphatase – increased
Blood antibody – titer increase
Blood bilirubin – increased
Blood IgG-specific antibodies – present
Blood IgM-specific antibodies – present
Blood liver enzymes – increased
Blood WBC – increased (leukocytosis)
Blood WBC – left shift

ECG

NS in absence of complications

Imaging

Lungs, parenchyma – consolidation [6]
Lungs, parenchyma – infiltrates (miliary)
Lungs, pleura – fluid (effusion)
Lungs – atelectasis

Other Tests

NS in absence of complications

Treatment – Nonpharmacologic

NS

Treatment – Pharmacologic

Antibiotics
        Doxycycline
        Erythromycin
        Tetracycline

Treatment – Surgical/Invasive

NA

Precautions

Laboratory handling of *chlamydia psittaci* organism ▲
Standard

Primary Prevention

Vaccine: no

Purchase and care of pet birds

Course

Symptom remission in 2-3 days with antibiotic treatment

Notes

[1]   Late in course
[2]   May initially present in coma
[3]   Severe, diffuse
[4]   Appearance of jaundice is rare and a poor prognostic sign
[5]   Horder's spots; resembles typhoid fever
[6]   Most common finding
[7]   Caution handling specimens ▲
[8]   Disseminated intravascular coagulation, placentitis

http://www.argus1.com/?psit

Updates

_____
_____
_____
_____
_____
_____
_____
_____
_____
_____
_____
_____
_____
_____
_____
_____
_____
_____
_____

Q Fever

Weapon
CDC Bioterrorism Category: B

Alternate Names
Query fever

Etiology
Coxiella burnetii [12]

Transmission
Source:	Infected dust and other materials from many animals, including sheep, cattle, goats, rodents, ticks [15]
Entry:	Contact
	Inhalation
Human-to-Human:	Rare

Predisposing/Comorbid Conditions
Cigarette smoking?

Demographics
Location:	Global
Populations:	All, esp slaughterhouse workers and veterinarians
Calendar:	Year-round

Systems
Liver/Biliary tract/Pancreas
Musculoskeletal
Nervous
Optic
Respiratory – lower [5, 9]

Incubation
1-4 weeks

Signs/Symptoms [8, 9, 10]

Abdomen, RUQ – pain
Appetite – decreased (anorexia)
Bowel movements – diarrhea
Chest – crackles (rales)
Chest – friction rub
Chest – pain, pleuritic
Chills
Cough, nonproductive
Eyes, retroorbital – pain
Eyes, vision – double (diplopia)
Face, unilat – pain
Fatigue
Head – pain (headache) [16]
Joints – pain (arthralgia)
Liver – large (hepatomegaly)
Mentation – hallucinations [3]
Mentation – weak (malaise)
Muscles – pain (myalgia)
Nausea
Neck, post – stiff (meningismus)
Skin, color – yellow (jaundice)
Skin – rash, macular [4]
Speech – disturbed (dysphasia)
Speech – inarticulate (dysarthria)
Spleen – large (splenomegaly)
Sweating – increased (hyperhydrosis)
Temperature, body – increased (fever)
Throat – sore
Vomiting
Weight – loss

Differentiation

Includes, but not limited to:

Brucellosis
Hepatitis
Influenza
Legionnaires' disease
Malaria

Other causes of pneumonia
Salmonellosis
Tularemia

Complications

Include, but not limited to:
Encephalomyelitis
Hepatitis
Infectious endocarditis [1]
Myocarditis
Optic neuritis
Osteomyelitis
Pericarditis

Laboratory [11] ▲

Blood culture – positive
Blood liver enzymes – increased
Blood platelets – decreased (thrombocytopenia) [7]
Blood serology – positive
Blood WBC – increased (leukocytosis)

ECG

NA in absence of complications

Imaging

Lungs, parenchyma – infiltrates [14]
Lungs, parenchyma – consolidation [14]
Lungs, pleura – fluid

Other Tests

Liver biopsy – granulomas, inflammation

Treatment – Nonpharmacologic

NS

Treatment – Pharmacologic

Antibiotics
Chloramphenicol
Quinolones

Rifampin
Tetracycline

Treatment – Surgical/Invasive
NA in absence of complications

Precautions
Laboratory handling of samples [11] ▲
Standard

Primary Prevention
Vaccine: yes [13]
Pasteurization

Course
Most cases resolve spontaneously

Notes
[1]   Esp aortic valve, prosthetic valve
[2]   Highly infective in humans
[3]   Auditory and visual
[4]   Erythematous, transient
[5]   Lungs – focal intraaveolar and bronchial necrosis
[6]   Granulomatous inflammation of liver and bones
[7]   Transient
[8]   Onset sudden
[9]   Pneumonia in about 50% of patients
[10]   50% or more of infected persons have no clinical illness
[11]   BSL-3 procedures ▲
[12]   Gram neg rod
[13]   For persons at high risk
[14]   Predilection for lower lobes
[15]   Transmitted among animals by ticks
[16]   May be severe
[17]   Usually normal

http://www.argus1.com/?qfever

Updates

_____

_____

_____

_____

_____

_____

_____

_____

_____

_____

_____

_____

_____

_____

_____

_____

_____

_____

_____

_____

Rift Valley Fever

Weapon
CDC Bioterrorism Category: A

Alternate Names
NA

Etiology
Bunyaviridae virus (genus *phlebovirus*)

After innoculation, virus replicates at exposure site, then migrates to target organ(s), mainly liver

Transmission
Source:	Mosquitoes and livestock, esp sheep
Entry:	Bite of mosquito and maybe fly
	Contact with blood/tissue of infected animals
Human-to-Human:	No

Predisposing/Comorbid Conditions
Skin abrasion

Demographics
Location:	Africa, Arabian peninsula
Populations:	Livestock workers, veterinarians, anyone exposed to mosquitoes in endemic area
Calendar:	Year-round

Systems
Coagulation
Liver/Biliary tract/Pancreas
Nervous
Optic
Skin

Incubation
2-6 days

Signs/Symptoms [3]
Abdomen, epigastrium – pain
Appetite – decreased (anorexia)
Back – pain
Bowel movements – blood or black (hematochezia) (melena)
Chills
Eyes, conjunctivae – injected
Eyes, light sensitivity – increased (photophobia)
Eyes, retina – exudate
Eyes, retina – hemorrhage
Eyes, retina macula – swollen (macular edema)
Eyes, retina – vascular occlusion
Eyes, vision – blind spots (scotoma)
Eyes, vision – loss, subtotal
Face – flushed
Head – pain (headache)
Mentation – weak (malaise)
Mentation – sleepy (somnolence)
Muscles – pain (myalgia)
Neck, post – stiff (meningismus)
Nose – blood (epistaxis)
Sense of taste – decreased/absent
Skin color – yellow (jaundice)
Skin – rash, purpura
Temperature, body – elevated (fever)
Vomiting
Vomiting – blood (hematemesis)

Differentiation
Includes, but not limited to:
Other viral hemorrhagic fevers

Complications
Include, but not limited to:
Encephalitis
Intracranial hemorrhage
Liver necrosis
Permanent vision loss

Laboratory [2] ▲
Blood clotting time – increased
Blood platelets – decreased (thrombocytopenia)
Blood serology – positive
Blood WBC – decreased (leukopenia)
Blood WBC – left shift
CSF – pleocytosis

ECG
NA in absence of complications

Imaging
NA in absence of complications

Other Tests
NA in absence of complications

Treatment – Nonpharmacologic
NS

Treatment – Pharmacologic
Ribavirin [1]

Treatment – Surgical/Invasive
NA in absence of complications

Precautions
BSL-3 or BSL-4 procedures ▲
Standard

Primary Prevention
Vaccine: experimental
Avoid sick animals in endemic areas
Mosquito control

Course
Overall mortality – 1%
Up to 50% mortality in patients with hemorrhagic syndrome ☠

Notes

[1]   Efficacy unproven
[2]   BSL-3 or BSL-4 procedures ▲
[3]   Infections often subclinical

http://argus1.com/?rift

Updates

_____
_____
_____
_____
_____
_____
_____
_____
_____
_____
_____
_____
_____
_____
_____
_____
_____
_____
_____
_____

Rocky Mountain Spotted Fever

Weapon
No [10]

Alternate Names
NA

Etiology
Rickettsia rickettsii

Infection of vascular endothelial cells causes multiple abnormal organ manifestations

Transmission
Source:	Ticks
Entry:	Tick bite [9]
	Inhalation (laboratory exposure)
Human-to-Human:	No

Predisposing/Comorbid Conditions
Increased morbidity and mortality with
  Advanced age
  African-American ethnicity
  Chronic alcohol abuse
  G6PD deficiency
  Male gender

Demographic
Location:	Western hemisphere
Populations:	All
Calendar:	Year-round, peak April-September

Systems

Coagulation
Liver/Biliary tract/Pancreas
Musculoskeletal
Nervous
Optic
Otic
Skin

Incubation

5-10 days

Signs/Symptoms

Abdomen – distention
Abdomen – pain [1]
Abdomen – tender
Appetite – decreased (anorexia)
Arterial pressure – low [2]
Arterial pulse, amplitude – decreased [2]
Back – stiff
Back, sacrum – swelling
Bowel movements – diarrhea
Bowel sounds – decreased/absent (ileus, adynamic)
Chills
Consciousness – loss, prolonged (coma) [2]
Cough – nonproductive
Ears, hearing – loss (deafness)
Eyes, conjunctivae – injected
Eyes, retina – petechiae
Eyes, vision – light sensitivity, increased (photophobia)
Extremities, ankles – swollen (edema)
Extremities, feet – swollen (edema)
Extremities, hands – swollen (edema)
Face – swelling
Head – pain (headache) [3]
Joints – pain (arthralgia)
Liver – enlargement (hepatomegaly)
Lymph nodes, gen – enlarged (lymphadenopathy)
Mood – lethargic, slowed
Mood – restless, irritable

Muscles – movement, slow spontaneous (athetosis)
Muscles – pain (myalgia) [4]
Muscles – rigid
Muscles – tender
Nausea
Neck – stiff (meningismus)
Seizures
Skin – dry
Skin – rash, macular [6]
Skin – rash, petechiae [5, 7]
Skin – ulcers
Sleep – disturbed (insomnia)
Spleen – enlarged (splenomegaly)
Temperature, body – elevated (fever)
Vomiting

Differentiation
Includes, but not limited to:
Ehrlichiosis
Infectious mononucleosis
Measles
Meningococcemia
Murine typhus
Rickettsialpox
Sepsis
Thrombotic thrombocytopenia purpura
Vasculitis

Complications
Include, but not limited to:
Acute respiratory distress syndrome (ARDS)
Cardiac dysrhythmias
Encephalitis
Gangrene of extremity
Hemiplegia
Myocarditis
Noncardiac pulmonary edema
Otitis media
Parotitis
Peripheral neuritis
Pnuemonia
Renal failure

Laboratory [8] ▲
Blood bilirubin – increased
Blood Hgb, Hct – decreased (anemia)
Blood liver enzymes – increased
Blood platelets, total – decreased (thrombocytopenia)
Blood serology – positive/rising titer
Blood sodium – decreased

ECG
NA in absence of complications

Imaging
NA in absence of complications

Other Tests
NA in absence of complications

Treatment – Nonpharmacologic
NS

Treatment – Pharmacologic
Doxycycline

Treatment – Surgical/Invasive
NA in absence of complications

Precautions [8]
Standard

Primary Prevention
Vaccine: no
Avoid tick-infested areas
Clothing barriers
Tick removal [11]

Course
Mortality untreated – 20% ☠

Notes

[1]   Abdominal muscles
[2]   Advanced cases
[3]   Excruciating, usually frontal
[4]   Esp back, legs
[5]   Esp over bony prominences
[6]   Begins 6 days or later after onset of symptoms, initially over wrists, ankles, palms, soles, forearms, then spreads centrally; occurs in 35–60% of patients
[7]   Increased by taking BP in an extremity (Rumpel – Leede phenomenon)
[8]   Precaution handling specimens ▲
[9]   Painless and often unnoticed
[10]   *Rickettsia rickettsii* has, however, been listed as a "select agent" under the USA Patriot Act
[11]   Includes finger protection, disinfection of bite site, avoid puncturing tick body

http://www.argus1.com/?rsmf

Updates

_____
_____
_____
_____
_____
_____
_____
_____
_____
_____
_____
_____
_____
_____
_____
_____
_____
_____
_____
_____
_____
_____

Rubella – Acquired

Weapon
No

Alternate Names
German measles
Third disease

Etiology
Togavirus, genus *rubivirus*

Replicates in nasopharynx and regional lymph nodes followed by viremia, when virus may cross placental barrier in pregnant women, causing fetal congenital rubella

Transmission
Source: Respiratory secretions [5]
Entry: Inhalation
Human-to-Human: Yes

Predisposing/Comorbid Conditions
NA

Demographics
Location: Global
Populations: All [1]
Calendar: Year-round, peak in spring

Systems
Lymphatic
Musculoskeletal
Skin

Incubation
12-23 days

Signs/Symptoms [6]

Appetite – decreased (anorexia)
Eyes, conjunctivae – injected
Head – pain (headache)
Joints – pain (arthralgia) [3]
Joints – stiffness [3]
Lymph nodes, postauricular – enlarged [2]
Lymph nodes, postcervical – enlarged
Lymph nodes, suboccipital – enlarged
Lymph nodes, gen – enlarged
Lymph nodes, gen – tender
Mentation – weakness (malaise)
Mouth, palate – Forscheimer's spots [7]
Mouth, palate – injected
Nose – drainage (rhinorrhea, coryza)
Skin – rash, macular/papular [4]
Skin – rash, pruritic [4]
Skin – rash, punctate [4]
Spleen – enlarged (splenomegaly)
Temperature, body – elevated (fever)
Testicles, bilateral – pain

Differentiation

Includes, but not limited to:

Drug rash
Erythema infectiosum
Infectious mononucleosis
Other viral exanthems
Parvovirus B19
Rubeola
Scarlet fever
Secondary syphilis
Toxoplasmosis

Complications

Include, but not limited to:

Arthritis
Congenital rubella
Encephalitis
Fetal infection

Hemorrhage
Hepatitis
Neuritis
Orchitis
Otitis media
Panencephalitis
Thrombocytopenia
Thrombocytopenic purpura

Laboratory
Blood lymphocytes – atypical
Blood platelets – decreased (thrombocytopenia)
Blood serology – positive
Blood WBC – decreased (leukopenia)

Imaging
NA

Other Tests
NA

Treatment – Nonpharmacologic
NS

Treatment – Pharmacologic
NS

Treatment – Surgical/Invasive
NA

Precautions
Standard

Primary Prevention
Vaccine: yes

Course
Recovery usual

Notes

[1]   Adults tend to be more ill

[2]   Highly characteristic

[3]   Very common in adult women; occurs with rash and may persist up to 1 month

[4]   Begins on face, then progresses downward; lasts about 3 days

[5]   10 days before to 15 days after rash appears

[6]   Often subclinical

[7]   Pinpoint petechiae and red macules

http://www.argus1.com/?rubella

Updates

_____

_____

_____

_____

_____

_____

_____

_____

_____

_____

_____

_____

_____

_____

_____

_____

_____

_____

_____

_____

Rubeola

Weapon
No

Alternate Names
Measles

Etiology
Measles virus, genus *morbillivirus*, family *paramyxoviridae*

Invades and multiplies in respiratory epithelium from nose to lungs; spreads via bloodstream leukocytes to reticulendothelial cells throughout body and to entire respiratory tract

Transmission
Source: Respiratory secretions from infected humans
Entry: Inhalation
Human-to-Human: Yes [9]

Predisposing/Comorbid Conditions
Increased severity in pregnant women and persons with immune deficiency or malnutrition

Demographics
Location: Global [10]
Populations: All, esp children
Calendar: Year-round with winter peak

Systems
Respiratory – lower
Respiratory – upper
Skin

Incubation

10-14 days

Signs/Symptoms

Abdomen – pain [6]
Abdomen, RLQ – pain [1]
Appetite – decreased (anorexia) [8]
Bowel movements – diarrhea
Cough – nonproductive
Eyes, conjunctivae – injected [8]
Eyes, vision – light sensitivity, increased (photophobia) [8]
Face – edema
Liver – enlarged (hepatomegaly) [2]
Lymph nodes, posterior cervical – enlarged
Mentation – weak (malaise) [8]
Mouth, mucosa – Koplick's spots [3]
Nose – drainage (rhinorrhea, coryza) [8]
Skin – rash, desquamating
Skin – rash, ecchymotic
Skin – rash, macular/papular [4]
Skin – rash, petechiae
Skin – rash, pruritic [5]
Spleen – enlarged (splenomegaly)
Temperature, body – elevated (fever) [8]
Vomiting

Differentiation

Includes, but not limited to:

Other causes of upper and lower respiratory tract infection
Other infectious and noninfectious causes of maculopapular rash

Complications

Include, but not limited to:

Bronchiolitis
Meningoencephalitis
Myocarditis
Otitis media
Pneumonia – bacterial [7]
Pneumonia – viral [7]
Spontaneous abortion

Subacute sclerosing panencephalitis [13]
Tuberculosis exacerbation/worsening

Laboratory

Blood serology – positive
Blood WBC – decreased (leukopenia)

ECG

NA

Imaging

NA in absence of complications

Other Tests

NA in absence of complications

Treatment – Nonpharmacologic

NS

Treatment – Pharmacologic

NS [11]

Treatment – Surgical/Invasive

NA

Precautions

Standard

Primary Prevention

Vaccine: yes
Immunoglobulin for exposure [12]

Course

Recovery usual

Notes

[1]   Due to involvement of appendix
[2]   Transient hepatitis, esp adults
[3]   Pathognomonic gray-white dots with red areolae, sometimes hemor-
      rhagic on buccal mucosa; may also occur on lower lip, palate

[4]   Begins on upper lateral and posterior neck, behind ears, along hair-
       line; spreads downward, reaching feet by 2-3 days
[5]   Usually mild
[6]   Due to mesenteric adenopathy
[7]   Primary measles or secondary bacterial
[8]   Prodromal phase
[9]   Highly infectious
[10]   Marked reduction in countries employing mass vaccinations
[11]   Oral vitamin A may be given to children to reduce morbidity and
       mortality in areas in which vitamin A deficiency is endemic
[12]   For persons at high risk for severe infections, i.e., HIV-positive
       persons, patients with cancer, etc
[13]   Many years after rubeola infection

http://www.argus1.com/?rubeola

Updates

Salmonellosis

Weapon
CDC Bioterrorism Category: B

Alternate Names
Nontyphoidal *salmonella*

Etiology
Salmonella enterica (*S enteritidis*)

Transmisission
Source: Humans and many domestic and wild animals
Entry: Ingestion of contaminated food
Human-to-Human: Yes (fecal-oral)

Predisposing/Comorbid Conditions
AIDS
Altered GI flora
Bartonellosis
Decreased gastric acidity
Decreased gastric motility
Diabetes mellitus
GI surgery
Hemolytic diseases
Histoplasmosis
Inflammatory bowel disease
Lymphoproliferative diseases
Malaria
Schistosomiasis

Demographics

Location:	Global
Populations:	All, esp very young, elderly, residents of institutions
Calendar:	Year-round

Systems

Gastrointestinal
Nervous

Incubation

6-72 hours

Signs/Symptoms [3]

Abdomen – distention [2]
Abdomen – pain [1]
Abdomen – tender [1]
Appetite – decreased (anorexia)
Bowel movements – diarrhea
Bowel sounds – increased
Head – pain (headache)
Mentation – confusion [2]
Mood – lethargy [2]
Nausea
Seizures [2]
Temperature, body – elevated (fever)
Vomiting

Differentiation

Includes, but not limited to:
Encephalitis
Other gastroenteritides

Complications

Include, but not limited to:
Arthritis – septic
Cholecystitis
Dehydration
Endocarditis
Extra-intestinal abscess
Meningitis

Osteomyelitis
Pericarditis
Reiter's syndrome
Septicemia
Toxic megacolon

Laboratory
Blood WBC – increased (leukocytosis) [4]
Stool blood – positive
Stool culture – positive
Stool WBC – positive

ECG
NA in absence of complications

Imaging
NA in absence of complications

Other Tests
NA in absence of complications

Treatment – Nonpharmacologic
Fluids and electrolytes

Treatment – Pharmacologic
Antibiotics for extra-intestinal spread

Treatment – Surgical/Invasive
NA in absence of complications

Precautions
Standard

Primary Prevention
Vaccine: no
Proper food handling and cooking

Course
Spontaneous resolution – 5-7 days

Notes

[1]   Esp periumbilcal area and RLQ
[2]   Part of severe form in some children; fever may be particularly high
[3]   Onset may be sudden
[4]   Usually mild or may be normal
[5]   Esp with sickle cell anemia, immune deficiency

http://www.argus1.com/?salmonella

Updates

_____
_____
_____
_____
_____
_____
_____
_____
_____
_____
_____
_____
_____
_____
_____
_____
_____
_____
_____

SARS

Weapon
No

Alternate Names
Severe acute respiratory syndrome

Etiology
SARS-associated coronavirus (SARS-CoV)

Transmission
Source:	Humans
	Contact
	Fecal-oral (possible)
Entry:	Inhalation
Human-to-Human:	Yes

Predisposing/Comorbid Conditions
Recent close contact with SARS patient or patient with severe respiratory illness who may have had contact with disease

Recent travel to domestic or foreign location with identified cases of SARS

Demographics
Location:	Global
Populations:	All, esp healthcare workers
Calendar:	Year-round

Systems
Respiratory – lower

Incubation
2-7 days

Signs/Symptoms [1]
Appetite – decreased (anorexia)
Bowel movements – diarrhea

Breathing – diff, rest (rest dyspnea)
Breathing – rapid (tachypnea)
Cough – nonproductive
Dizziness (lightheaded)
Head – pain (headache)
Mentation – confusion
Mentation – weak (malaise)
Muscles – pain (myalgia)
Muscles – stiffness
Nose, drainage – increased (rhinorrhea, coryza) [2]
Temperature, body – elevated (fever)
Throat – sore [2]

Differentiation
Includes, but not limited to:
Acute respiratory distress syndrome (ARDS)
Pneumonia

Complications
Include, but not limited to:
Acute respiratory distress syndrome (ARDS)

Laboratory [4] ▲
Blood C-reactive protein (CRP) – increased
Blood creatine kinase (CK) – increased
Blood liver enzymes – increased
Blood lymphocytes – decreased (lymphopenia)
Blood platelets – decreased (thrombocytopenia)
Blood partial thromboplastin time (PTT) – increased
Blood serology – positive [3]

ECG
NA in absence of complications

Imaging
Lungs, parenchyma general – infiltrates

Other Tests
Arterial blood gases

Treatment – Nonpharmacologic
Respiratory support

Treatment – Pharmacologic

NS

Treatment – Surgical/Invasive

NA in absence of complications

Precautions

Air and contact barriers ▲
Standard

Primary Prevention

Vaccine: no
Avoid contact
Avoid travel to areas with active infection
Isolation of cases ▲

Course

Variable
Fatal in 5% of cases

Notes

[1] Chest signs may be strikingly normal in contrast to radiographic changes
[2] Usually absent
[3] CDC states that SARS-CoV antibody detection is best indicator of infection
[4] BSL-3 procedures ▲

http://www.argus1.com/?sars

Updates

Shigellosis

Weapon
CDC Bioterrorism Category: B

Alternate Names
Bacillary dysentery

Etiology
S boydii
S dysenteriae
S flexneri
S sonnei

Transmission
Source:	Humans
Entry:	Ingestion
Human-to-Human:	Yes (fecal-oral)

Predisposing/Comorbid Conditions
Advanced age
Debilitation
Malnourishment

Demographic
Location:	Global
Populations:	All, esp persons living in crowded living conditions with poor hygienic conditions, such as jails, day care centers, refugee camps; uncommon <age 6 months
Calendar:	Year-round

Systems
Gastrointestinal

Incubation
Usual – 1-3 days (range $1/2$-7 days)

Signs/Symptoms
Abdomen – distention
Abdomen – pain
Abdomen – tender
Anorectum – prolapse
Anorectum – tender
Appetite – decreased (anorexia)
Bowel movements, control – decreased/absent
Bowel movements, stool – blood or black (hematochezia) (melena)
Bowel movements, stool – mucoid
Bowel movements, stool – pustular
Bowel movements – diarrhea
Bowel movements – difficult/painful (tenesmus)
Bowel sounds – increased
Consciousness – loss, prolonged (coma) [1]
Mentation – delirium [1]
Mentation – weakness (malaise)
Mood – lethargy
Mood – restless/irritable
Nausea
Seizures [1]
Temperature, body – elevated (fever)
Vomiting

Differentiation
Includes, but not limited to:
Other gastroenteritides

Complications
Include, but not limited to:
Arthritis
Dehydration
Intestinal perforation
Myocarditis
Neuritis

Laboratory
Blood WBC – decreased (leukopenia) [2]
Blood WBC – increased (leukocytosis) [2]
Stool blood – positive
Stool culture – positive
Stool WBC – positive [4]

ECG
NA in absence of complications

Imaging
NA in absence of complications

Other tests
NA in absence of complications

Treatment – Nonpharmacologic
Fluids and electrolytes

Treatment – Pharmacologic
Antibiotics [3]
Cephalosporins
Fluoroquinolones
Avoid anti-diarrheal medications

Treatment – Surgical/Invasive
NA in absence of complications

Precautions
Enteric
Standard

Primary Prevention
Vaccine: no
Hygiene

Course
Variable
Spontaneous resolution usual in 1-6 weeks

Notes

[1] May occur in a rare form of *s dysenteriae* without diarrhea
[2] Leukocytosis with left shift usual
[3] Antibiotic selection should be made on case-by-case basis according to sensitivities because resistance is common
[4] Also present in other infectious enteritides and in ulcerative colitis

http://www.argus1.com/?shigella

Updates

_____
_____
_____
_____
_____
_____
_____
_____
_____
_____
_____
_____
_____
_____
_____
_____
_____
_____
_____

Smallpox

Weapon
CDC Bioterrorism Category: A

Alternate Names
Variola

Etiology
Variola virus, a DNA orthopoxvirus

Viral implantation into oropharynx/respiratory tract; spreads to regional lymph nodes; viremia with virus multiplication in spleen, bone marrow, lymph nodes; locates in leukocytes, small dermal blood vessels, and submucosal oral and pharyngeal cells

Transmission
Source:	Humans prior to global eradication; presently maintained only in laboratories
Entry:	Direct (person to person) – respiratory aerosol
	Indirect – contact with contaminated items
Human-to-Human:	Yes

Predisposing/Comorbid Conditions
Pregnancy – hemorrhagic form

Demographics
Location:	Global
Populations:	All; distribution probably similar to general population except for residual immunity from prior vaccination in older population
Calendar:	Year-round, peak winter and spring

Systems
Oropharynx
Skin

Incubation
7-17 days

Signs/Symptoms
Abdomen – pain [1]
Back – pain [13]
Bowel movements – diarrhea
Chills
Cough
Head – pain (headache) [13]
Mentation – delirium
Mentation – weak (malaise) [13]
Mouth, mucosa – hemorrhage [h]
Mouth, mucosa – petechiae
Mouth, mucosa – pustules [21]
Mouth, mucosa – ulcers [21]
Mouth, mucosa – vesicles [21]
Nausea
Prostration [h] [m] [13]
Skin, color gen – red (erythema) [h] [17]
Skin – rash, hemorrhagic [h]
Skin – rash, macular/papular [3, 9, 12, 14, 17]
Skin – rash, petechiae [h]
Skin – rash, pustular [3, 7, 11, 12, 14, 17]
Skin – rash, vesicular [3, 12, 14, 17]
Skin – scarring, residual [8]
Temperature, body – elevated (fever) [13]
Throat – maculopapular lesions
Throat – petechiae
Throat – pustules
Throat – ulcers
Throat – vesicles
Vomiting [13]

Differentiation
Includes, but not limited to:
Acute abdomen [h] [m]

Chickenpox [10]
Cowpox [2]
Drug erruption
Hand, foot, and mouth disease
Herpes zoster, disseminated
Leukemia – acute
Measles
Meningococcemia
Molluscum contagiosum
Monkeypox [2]
Rickettsialpox
Syphylis, secondary
Vaccinia
Variola minor

Complications
Include, but not limited to:
Bacterial secondary infections [15]
Blepharitis
Conjunctivitis
Corneal ulceration/keratitis
Dehydration/hypovolemia
Encephalitis
Hemorrhage [16]
Myocarditis
Noncardiac pulmonary edema
Orchitis
Osteomyelitis variolosa
Pneumonia
Shock

Laboratory [19] ▲
Skin fluid EM – virons present [18]
Exclusion of varicella zoster virus (DFA, EM, polymerase chain reaction)

ECG
NA in absence of complications

Imaging
NA in absence of complications

Other Tests
NA in absence of complications

Treatment – Nonpharmacologic
NS

Treatment – Pharmacologic
NS

Treatment – Surgical/Invasive
NA in absence of complications

Precautions
Airborne [22]
BSL-4 procedures ▲
Contact [22]
Droplet [22]
Standard [22]

Primary Prevention
Vaccine: yes [20]
Quarantine

Course
Mortality, hemorrhagic and malignant forms – usually fatal ☠
Mortality, usual form – 30% [5] ☠

Notes
[h]	Hemorrhagic form
[m]	Malignant form
[1]	Can be predominant symptom leading to mistaken exploratory surgery in malignant form
[2]	Uncommonly transmitted person-to-person
[3]	Area lesions at same stage of development are well-circumscribed; chickenpox lesions present at all stages and less demarcated
[4]	Within 4 days of exposure
[5]	Course more benign among prior vaccinated persons
[7]	Round, tense, deeply imbedded
[8]	Face most severe
[9]	Begins on face, hands, forearms, followed by trunk
[10]	Unlike smallpox, rash often begins on trunk with lesions present in all stages

[11] Malignant form does not progress to this stage, with lesions remaining soft and flat

[12] Lesions progress much more slowly than chickenpox

[13] Febrile prodrome before rash is highly characteristic; fever is high and other symptoms present

[14] May occur on palms and soles, which is unusual in chickenpox

[15] Skin, joints, septicemia

[16] If severe, disseminated intravascular coagulation should be considered

[17] Rash has more centripetal distribution than chickenpox, which is more prominent on trunk

[18] Brick shape; in vesicular and pustular fluid

[19] BSL-4 procedures ▲

[20] Within 7 days after exposure prevents or lessens infection severity

[21] Oral lesions signify beginning of contagium

[22] Until all scabs separated

http://www.argus1.com/?smallpox

Updates

_____
_____
_____
_____
_____
_____
_____
_____
_____
_____
_____
_____
_____
_____
_____
_____

Staphylococcus Food Poisoning

Weapon
CDC Bioterrorism Category: B

Alternate Names
NA

Etiology
Staphylococcus enterotoxin B

Transmission
Source:	Contaminated foods left at room temperature
Entry:	Ingestion
Human-to-Human:	No

Predisposing/Comorbid Conditions
NA

Demographics
Location:	Global
Populations:	All
Calendar:	Year-round

Systems
Gastrointestinal

Incubation
2-8 hours

Signs/Symptoms
Abdomen – pain
Bowel movements, stool – blood or black (hematochezia) (melena)

Bowel movements, stool – mucoid
Bowel movements – diarrhea
Nausea
Temperature, body – elevated (fever) [1]
Vomiting

Differentiation
Includes, but not limited to:
Other forms of gastroenteritis

Complications
Include, but not limited to:
Dehydration

Laboratory
Blood concentration – increased (hemoconcentration)

ECG
NA in absence of complications

Imaging
NA in absence of complications

Other Tests
Isolate coagulase-positive staph from food source

Treatment – Nonpharmacologic
Fluids and electrolytes

Treatment – Pharmacologic
Antidiarrheals
Antiemetics

Treatment – Surgical/Invasive
NA in absence of complications

Precautions
NA

Primary Prevention
Proper food storage and preparation

Course
3-6 hours
Recovery usual

Note
[1]　Uncommon

http://www.argus1.com/?staphfood

Updates

_____
_____
_____
_____
_____
_____
_____
_____
_____
_____
_____
_____
_____
_____
_____
_____
_____
_____
_____
_____

Streptococcal Pharyngitis

Weapon
No

Alternate Names
Strep throat

Etiology
Group A streptococci [7]

Transmission
Source: Humans
Entry: Direct oral/throat contact with infected secretions
                           Ingestion of contaminated food, esp milk products [5]
                           Inhalation
Human-to-Human: Yes

Predisposing/Comorbid Conditions
NA

Demographics
Location: Global
Populations: All, esp school-age children
Calendar: Year-round with winter-spring peak

Systems
Lymphatic
Oropharynx

Incubation
1-3 days

Signs/Symptoms

Abdomen, gen – pain
Chills
Head – pain (headache)
Heart rate – increased (tachycardia)
Lymph nodes, ant cervical – enlarged
Lymph nodes, submaxillary – enlarged
Lymph nodes, tonsillar – enlarged
Lymph nodes, tonsillar – exudate
Mentation – weak (malaise)
Mouth, palate – petechiae
Nausea
Nose, drainage – increased (rhinorrhea, coryza) [1]
Temperature, body – elevated (fever)
Throat – exudate
Throat – injected
Throat – sore
Vomiting

Differentiation [2]

Includes, but not limited to:
A hemolyticum
Brucellosis
Diphtheria
Infectious mononucleosis
Mycoplasma
Neisseria gonorrheae
Neisseria meningitidis
Salmonellosis
Tonsillar tuberculosis
Toxoplasmosis
Tularemia
Viral pharyngitis
Yersiniosis

Complications

Include, but not limited to:
Acute glomerulonephritis
Acute rheumatic fever
Bronchopneumonia [3]
Cervical adenitis [3]

Endocarditis [4]
Mastoiditis [3]
Meningitis [4]
Osteomyelitits [4]
Otitis media [3]
Parapharyngeal abscess [3]
Retropharyngeal abscess [3]
Scarlet fever
Septic arthritis [4]
Sinusitis [3]

Laboratory
Blood CRP – increased
Blood WBC – increased (leukocytosis)
Throat culture – positive
Throat rapid antigen detection – positive

ECG
NA in absence of complications [6]

Imaging
NA in absence of complications

Other Tests
NA in absence of complications

Treatment – Nonpharmacologic
NS

Treatment – Pharmacologic
Antibiotics
    Penicillin
    Erythromycin [8]

Treatment – Surgical/Invasive
NA in absence of complications

Precautions
Standard

Primary Prevention
Vaccine: no

Food handling
Hygiene
Pasteurization

Course

Treated – 1-3 days
Untreated – 2-5 days

Notes

[1]   Children under 4; may be only symptom in this age group – otherwise
      this symptom suggests another etiology, esp viral
[2]   All causes of acute pharyngitis
[3]   Direct extension
[4]   Hematogenous spread
[5]   May cause sudden community-wide outbreak
[6]   May be abnormal if acute rheumatic fever occurs as complication
[7]   Other serogroups, esp C and G, sometimes cause
[8]   If allergic to penicillin

http://www.argus1.com/?strepphar

Updates

Trichinellosis

Weapon
No

Alternate Names
Trichiniasis
Trichinosis

Etiology
Trichinella spiralis

Transmission
Source: Domestic and wild animals [2]
Entry: Ingestion of *trichinella* cysts in under-cooked meat
Human-to-Human: No

Predisposing/Comorbid Conditions
NA

Demographics
Location: Global
Populations: All
Calendar: Year-round

Systems
Cardiovascular
Gastrointestinal
Musculoskeletal
Optic
Respiratory – lower
Skin

Incubation

Intestinal phase – 1-2 days

Systemic phase – 2-8 weeks

Signs/Symptoms [7]

Abdomen – cramps [1]

Abdomen – distention [1]

Abdomen – pain [1]

Appetite – decreased (anorexia) [1]

Bowel movements – constipation [1]

Bowel movements – diarrhea [1]

Breathing – diff, effort (effort dyspnea) [1]

Breathing – diff, rest (rest dyspnea) [5, 6]

Chest – pain, pleuritic [3, 5]

Chills [1, 3]

Cough – nonproductive [3]

Extremities, hands/nails – hemorrhage [3]

Eyes, conjunctivae/bulba/peri-cornea – swollen (chemosis) [3]

Eyes, conjunctivae – hemorrhage [3]

Eyes, conjunctivae – injected [3]

Eyes, light sensitivity – increased (photophobia) [3]

Eyes, retina – hemorrhage [3]

Eyes, surrounding tissue – swollen (periorbital edema) [3]

Eyes – pain [3]

Face – swollen [3]

Head – pain (headache)

Mentation – weak (malaise) [1, 3]

Mouth, chewing – pain [3]

Muscles, back – pain [3]

Muscles, extremities/upper proximal – pain [3]

Muscles, jaw – pain [3]

Muscles, local – swollen [3]

Muscles, local – tender [3]

Muscles, neck – pain [3]

Muscles – hard [3]

Muscles – pain (myalgia) [3, 14]

Muscles – stiff [3]

Nausea [1]

Skin – rash, macular [1, 3]

Skin – rash, petechiae [1, 3]

Swallowing – pain (odynophagia) [3]
Sweating – increased (hyperhydrosis) [1, 3]
Temperature, body – elevated (fever) [1, 3]
Thirst –increased [3]
Tongue – large (macroglossia) [3]
Tongue – pain [3]
Tongue – tender (glossitis) [3]
Vomiting [1]

Differentiation
Includes, but not limited to:
Angioedema
Gastroenteritis
Other intestinal parasitic infections
Polyarteritis nodosa
Polymyositis
Typhoid fever

Complications
Include, but not limited to:
Congestive heart failure
Meningoencephalitis
Myocarditis
Pneumonitis
Respiratory failure

Laboratory
Blood creatine kinase (CK) – increased [13]
Blood eosinophiles – increased (eosinophilia)
Blood IgE – increased
Blood serology – positive [8]
Blood troponin – increased [9]
Blood WBC – increased (leukocytosis)

ECG
NA in absence of complications [9]

Imaging
NA in absence of complications

Other Tests
Electromyogram [11]
Muscle biopsy [12]

Treatment – Nonpharmacologic
Analgesia [3]
Bed rest [3]

Treatment – Pharmacologic
Corticosteroids [3, 13]
Thiabendazole [1]

Treatment – Surgical/Invasive
NA in absence of complications

Precautions
NA

Primary Prevention
Vaccine: no
Adequate cooking of animal meat

Course
Recovery usual

Notes
[1]   Intestinal phase, usually lasts up to 7 days, weeks in some cases
[2]   Pork, bear, wild feline, fox, dog, wolf, horse, seal, walrus
[3]   Systemic phase
[4]   Esp jaw, neck, upper arm, lower back
[5]   Involvement of diaphragm and intercostal muscles
[6]   May progress to respiratory failure
[7]   Severity determined by infection bolus; usually subclinical
[8]   Week 2-3
[9]   I.e., myocarditis
[10]   For CNS, lung involvement
[11]   To differentiate from other myopathies
[12]   Only when definitive diagnosis required
[13]   Severe infections
[14]   May occur suddenly

http://www.argus1.com/?trich

Updates

_____
_____
_____
_____
_____
_____
_____
_____
_____
_____
_____
_____
_____
_____
_____
_____
_____
_____
_____
_____

Tularemia

Weapon
CDC Bioterrorism Category: A

Alternate Names
Anginose [op]
Deer-fly fever
Francis disease
Ohara fever
Rabbit fever

Etiology
Francisella tularensis [10]

Bacteria multiply in regional lymph nodes causing cell death, local release of bacteria, and systemic hematogenous dissemination

Transmission
Source:	Mainly wild animals; domestic animals; hard ticks in rodent-mosquito cycle in European and Asian northern latitudes
Entry:	Bites – arthropods, esp ticks in USA and mosquitoes in Scandinavia
	Contact – infected animal tissue, soil
	Ingestion – infected food, soil, water
	Inhalation – infected aerosol
Human-to-Human:	No

Predisposing/Comorbid Conditions
Skin abrasion

Demographics
Location:	Global; USA – rural, esp midwest
Populations:	All
Calendar:	Year-round, peak June-September

Systems

Liver/Biliary tract/Pancreas
Lymphatic
Optic
Oropharynx
Respiratory – lower
Skin

Incubation

3-14 days

Signs/Symptoms [1, 6]

Abdomen – pain
Appetite – decreased (anorexia)
Bowel movements – diarrhea [T]
Breathing, rest – difficult (rest dyspnea) [P]
Breathing – rapid (tachypnea) [P]
Chest, ant – pain/tightness/burning, nonpleuritic [P]
Chest – pain, pleuritic [P]
Chills
Cough – acute, NS [P]
Cough – nonproductive [P]
Cough – productive [P]
Eyes, conjunctiva/bulba/peri-cornea – swollen (chemosis) [OC] [2, 7]
Eyes, conjunctivae – injected [OC] [2]
Eyes, conjunctivae – purulent [OC] [2]
Eyes, conjunctivae – ulcers [OC] [2]
Eyes, lids – swelling (edema) [OC] [2]
Eyes, light sensitivity – increased (photophobia) [OC] [2]
Eyes, tears (lacrimation) – increased [OC] [2]
Eyes – pain [O] [2, 13]
Fatigue
Head – pain (headache)
Heart rate – decreased relative to temp (relative bradycardia)
Joints – pain (arthralgia)
Liver – enlarged (hepatomegaly)
Liver – tender
Lymph nodes, regional – enlarged [U] [OC][4, 7, 12]
Lymph nodes, regional – draining [U] [OC] [4, 12]
Lymph nodes, regional – tender [U] [OC] [4, 12]

Lymph nodes, tonsillar – enlarged [OP] [4]
Mentation – weak (malaise)
Mouth, mucosa – inflammation (stomatitis) [OP}
Mouth, mucosa – ulcers [OP]
Muscles – pain (myalgia)
Nausea
Nose, drainage – increased (rhinorhea, coryza)
Skin, extensor surfaces – nodes, painful (erythema nodosum)
Skin, single lesion – draining [U]
Skin, single lesion – macule/papule [U]
Skin, single lesion – painful, stinging [U]
Skin, single lesion – ulcer [U]
Spleen – enlarged (splenomegaly)
Spleen – tender
Sputum – blood (hemoptysis)
Sputum – purulent
Temperature, body – elevated (fever) [5]
Throat – exudate [OP]
Throat – sore [OP]
Vomiting
Weight – loss

Differentiation
Includes, but not limited to:
Atypical pneumonia
Bacterial pneumonia
Influenza
Other causes of infectious lymphadenopathy and dermopathy
Q fever

Complications
Include, but not limited to:
Disseminated intravascular coagulation
Endocarditis
Hepatitis
Lung abscess
Mediastinitis
Meningitis
Osteomyelitis
Pericarditis
Peritonitis
Pneumonia

Respiratory failure
Renal failure
Rhabdomyolysis [T]
Sepsis
Suppurative lymphadenopathy

Laboratory [9, 12] ▲

Blood creatine kinase (CK) – increased [T]
Blood platelets – decreased (thrombocytopenia)
Blood serology – positive
Blood sodium – decreased [T]
Blood WBC – increased (leukocytosis)
Body fluids, bacterial stain – positive
Body fluids, fluorescent antibody – positive
Tissue biopsy, bacterial culture – positive
Tissue biopsy, bacterial stain – positive
Urine myoglobin – positive (myoglobinuria)
Urine WBC – present

ECG

NA in absence of complications

Imaging

Lungs, hilar lymph nodes – enlarged
Lungs, parenchyma – infiltrates
Lungs, pleura – fluid

Other Tests

NS in absence of complications

Treatment – Nonpharmacologic

Fluids

Treatment – Pharmacologic

Antibiotics
Gentamycin
Streptomycin

Treatment – Surgical/Invasive

NA in absence of complications

Precautions

Handling body specimens ▲
Standard

Primary Prevention

Vaccine: yes [11]

Care when handling wildlife

Prophylactic antibiotics for high-risk exposure

Course – untreated

Variable

Mortality treated – ≤2%

Mortality untreated – 5-60% ☠

Notes

[OC]   Occuloglandular form

[OP]   Oropharyngeal form

[P]   Pulmonary form

[T]   Typhoidal form

[U]   Ulceroglandular form

[1]   Great overlap among different forms

[2]   Unilateral; part of Parinaud's syndrome

[3]   Epitrochlear, axillary nodes – rabbit bite; inguinal, femoral nodes – tick bite; preauricular, submandibular, cervical nodes – ocuoglandular form; mesenteric nodes – intestinal form

[4]   Glandular form if only lymph node enlargement occurs without other s/s present

[5]   If no other s/s present – "typhoidal" form

[6]   Onset abrupt

[7]   May be severe

[8]   Bubo

[9]   Level A laboratory procedures ▲

[10]   Aerobic gram-negative coccobacillus

[11]   For persons at high risk

[12]   Lab tests often normal

http://www.argus1.com/?tul

Updates

_____

_____

_____

_____

_____

_____

_____

Typhoid Fever

Weapon
No

Alternate Names
Enteric fever

Etiology
Salmonella typhi

After ingestion, *s syphi* invades intestinal wall and multiplies in lymphoid tissue (Peyer's patches) causing local tissue ulcers followed by bacteremia and infection of liver, spleen, bone marrow; secondary bacteremia causes infection in other sites including tumor, aneurysm, bone, gall bladder (in presence of galls stones) [2]

Transmission
Source:	Human
Entry:	Ingestion – food, water contaminated by infectious feces
Human-to-Human:	Yes

Predisposing/Comorbid Conditions
Achlorhydria
Biliary tract disease
Cancer, esp lymphoma
Immunodeficiency
Malnutrition
Reticuloendothelial abnormalities [3]
Urinary tract disease

Demographics
Location:	Global, esp tropics
Populations:	All
Calendar:	Year-round

Systems
Gastrointestinal
Hematopoietic/Immune
Liver/Biliary tract/Pancreas
Lymphatic

Incubation Period
5-21 days

Signs/Symptoms
Abdomen – pain [13]
Abdomen – tender [13]
Appetite – reduced (anorexia)
Behavior – bizarre or changed   [5]
Bowel movements – constipation
Bowel movements – diarrhea
Bowel sounds – increased
Breath sounds, gen – crackling (rales)
Chills
Cough – nonproductive
Dizziness – lightheaded
Eyes, conjunctivae – injected
Head – pain (headache)
Heart rate – slow relative to fever (relative bradycardia)
Joints – pain (arthralgia)
Liver – enlarged (hepatomegaly)
Lymph nodes, ant cervical – enlarged
Mentation – feeling of weakness (malaise)
Mentation – NS changes [4]
Muscles – pain (myalgia)
Nausea
Nose – blood (epistaxis)
Seizures
Skin – rash, macular [1]
Spleen – enlarged (splenomegaly)
Sweating – increased (hyperhydrosis)
Temperature, body – elevated (fever)
Throat – sore
Vomiting
Weight – loss

Differentiation
Includes, but not limited to:
 Causes of acute abdomen
 Leishmaniasis
 Malaria
 Meningoencephalitis [6]
 Other gastroenteritides

Complications
Include, but not limited to:
 Bowel perforation
 Endocarditis
 Local abscess
 Necrotizing cholecystitis
 Pancreatitis
 Pericarditis
 Seizures
 Spontaneous abortion

Laboratory
 Blood culture – positive
 Blood Hgb/Hct – decreased (anemia)
 Blood liver enzymes – increased
 Blood muscle enzymes – increased
 Blood platelets – decreased (thrombocytopenia)
 Blood serology – positive
 Blood WBC – decreased (leukopenia)
 Blood WBC – increased (leukocytosis)
 Bone marrow culture – positive [7]
 Skin bacterial culture – positive
 Stool culture – positive

ECG
 NS ST-T wave changes

Imaging
 NA in absence of complications

Other Tests
 Liver biopsy [8]

Treatment – Nonpharmacologic
NS

Treatment – Pharmacologic
Antibiotics [10]
      Cephalosporins
      Chloramphenicol [10]
      Fluroquinolones [9]
Corticosteroids [11]

Treatment – Surgical/Invasive
NA in absence of complications, i.e., bowel perforation

Precautions
Enteric
Standard

Primary Prevention
Vaccine: yes [12]
Hygiene

Course
Usually resolves with/without antibiotic treatment

Notes
[1]   "Rose spots" on abdomen – culture positive
[2]   Gallbladder infection leads to chronic carrier state
[3]   Sickle cell and other hemoglobinopathies, malaria, schistosomiasis, bartonellosis, histoplasmosis
[4]   Apathy, confusion, psychosis, etc.
[5]   I.e., picking at imaginary objects ("muttering delerium")
[6]   CSF normal in typhoid fever
[7]   Highly sensitive
[8]   Mononuclear cell infiltration, Kupffer cell hyperplasia
[9]   Probably drug class of choice unless resistance is present
[10]   Resistance common
[11]   Short-term, severe cases
[12]   Recommended for travelers to endemic areas of infection
[13]   May localize to RLQ and resemble acute appendicitis

http://www.argus1.com/?typhoid

Updates

_____

_____

_____

_____

_____

_____

_____

_____

_____

_____

_____

_____

_____

_____

_____

_____

_____

_____

_____

Typhus – Epidemic

Weapon
CDC Bioterrorism Category: B

Alternate Names
Brill-Zinsser disease [6]
Exanthematic typhus
Louse-borne tick fever
Sutama

Etiology
R. Prowazekii [9]

Endothelial cell necrosis causing vasculitis and abnormal blood clotting

Transmission
Source:	Body louse from infected humans
	Flying squirrels?
Entry:	Bite of body louse
	Inhalation
Human-to-Human:	Via louse

Predisposing/Comorbid Conditions
Malnourishment
Poor hygiene

Demographics
Location:	Global, esp mountains
Populations:	All, esp those in poor living conditions
Calendar:	Year-round

Systems
Coagulation
Gastrointestinal

Nervous
Optic
Otic
Respiratory – lower
Skin

Incubation

6-15 days

Signs/Symptoms [5]

Abdomen – pain
Abdomen – tender
Appetite – decreased (anorexia)
Arterial pressure – decreased
Back, lower (lumbar) – pain
Bowel movements – constipation
Bowel movements – diarrhea
Bowel sounds – decreased/absent (ileus, adynamic)
Breath sounds – crackles (rales) [1]
Chills
Consciousness – loss, prolonged (coma)
Cough – nonproductive
Ears, hearing – loss (deafness) [2]
Ears – dizziness/spinning (vertigo, true)
Ears – ringing (tinnitus)
Eyes, conjunctivae – injected
Eyes, retroorbital – pain
Eyes, vision – light sensitity, increased (photophobia)
Head – pain (headache) [3]
Heart rate – increased (tachycardia)
Heart rate – decreased relative to fever (bradycardia, relative)
Joints – pain (arthralgia)
Mentation – confusion
Mentation – delirium
Mentation – sleepy (somnolence)
Mentation – weak (malaise)
Mood – labile
Mood – lethargic
Mood – restless/irritable
Muscles – pain (myalgia) [10]

Muscles – weak
Nausea
Neck, post – stiff (meningismus)
Skin – rash, macular [4]
Spleen – enlarged (splenomegaly)
Sputum – blood (hemoptysis)
Temperature, body – elevated (fever)
Vomiting

Differentiation

Includes, but not limited to:
Acute abdomen
Malaria
Pneumonia
Relapsing fever
Tuberculosis

Complications

Include, but not limited to:
Cerebral infarction
Hypotension
Pneumonia
Renal failure
Skin gangrene

Laboratory

Blood complement fixation antibodies – positive
Blood creatinine – increased
Blood Hgb/Hct – decreased (anemia)
Blood liver enzymes – increased [7]
Blood platelets – decreased (thrombocytopenia)
Blood serology – positive [8]
Blood WBC – decreased (leukopenia) [7]
Blood WBC – increased (leukocytosis)
Urine RBC – present (hematuria, microhematuria)

ECG

NA in absence of complications

Imaging

Lungs, parenchyma – infiltrates

Other Tests
NA in absence of complications

Treatment – Nonpharmacologic
NS

Treatment – Pharmacologic
Antibiotics
> Chloramphenicol
> Doxycycline
> Tetracycline

Treatment – Surgical/Invasive
NA in absence of complications

Precautions
Standard

Primary Prevention
Vaccine: no
Eliminate lice in clothes and bedding
Exposure only – doxycycline

Course
Mortality – 10-60% ☠

Notes
[1]   Mainly bases
[2]   Transient
[3]   Esp frontal
[4]   Initially axillae and inner arm, then abdomen, shoulders, chest, thighs and becomes maculopapular
[5]   Similar to murine typhus, but more severe
[6]   Recurrence years after first episode, often older persons, usually milder form
[7]   Mild
[8]   *Proteus ox-19* agglutinins
[9]   Obligate intracellular gram-negative bacillus
[10]   May be severe

http://www.argus1.com/?tyepi

Updates

_____
_____
_____
_____
_____
_____
_____
_____
_____
_____
_____
_____
_____
_____
_____
_____
_____
_____
_____

Typhus – Murine

Weapon
No

Alternate Names
Endemic typhus fever

Etiology
Rickettsia typhi

Transmission
Source:	Rats, mice
Entry:	Flea bites
	Inhalation (uncommon)
Human-to-Human:	No

Predisposing/Comorbid Conditions
NA

Demographics
Location:	Global, esp coastal areas
Populations:	All
Calendar:	Peak summer-autumn

Systems
Gastrointestinal
Musculoskeletal
Nervous
Optic
Otic
Skin

Incubation

8-16 days

Signs/Symptoms [5]

Abdomen – pain

Appetite – decreased (anorexia)

Arterial pressure, gen – decreased

Back, lower (lumbar) – pain

Bowel movements – constipation

Bowel movements – diarrhea

Bowel sounds – decreased/absent (ileus, adynamic)

Breath sounds, gen – crackles (rales) [1]

Chills

Consciousness – loss, prolonged (coma)

Cough – nonproductive

Ears, hearing – loss (deafness) [2]

Ears – dizziness/spinning (vertigo, true)

Ears – ringing (tinnitus)

Eyes, conjunctivae – injected

Eyes, retroorbital – pain

Head – pain (headache) [3]

Heart rate – increased (tachycardia)

Heart rate – decreased relative to fever (bradycardia, relative)

Joints – pain (arthralgia)

Liver – enlarged (hepatomegaly)

Mentation – confusion

Mentation – delirium

Mentation – sleepy (somnolence)

Mentation – weak (malaise)

Mood – labile

Mood – lethargic

Mood – restless/irritable

Muscles – pain (myalgia)

Muscles – weak

Nausea

Neck, post – stiff (meningismus)

Skin – rash, macular [4]

Spleen – large (splenomegaly)

Sputum – blood (hemoptysis)

Temperature, body – elevated (fever)
Vomiting

Differentiation
Includes, but not limited to:
Encephalitis
Epidemic typhus
Rocky Mountain spotted fever

Complications
Include, but not limited to:
Circulatory failure
Renal failure
Respiratory failure

Laboratory
Blood calcium – decreased
Blood liver enzymes – increased
Blood platelets – decreased (thrombocytopenia)
Blood serology – positive
Blood WBC – decreased (leukopenia)
Blood WBC – increased (leukocytosis)

ECG
NA in absence of complications

Imaging
NA in absence of complications

Other Tests
NA in absence of complications

Treatment – Nonpharmacologic
NS

Treatment – Pharmacologic
Antibiotics
Chloramphenicol
Doxycycline
Tetracycline

Treatment – Surgical/Invasive
NA in absence of complications

Precautions
Standard

Primary Prevention
Vaccine: no
Flea/Rodent control

Course
Mortality <1%

Notes
[1]   Mainly bases
[2]   Transient
[3]   Esp frontal
[4]   Trunk, extremities
[5]   Similar to epidemic typhus, but less severe

http://www.argus1.com/?tymur

Updates

_____
_____
_____
_____
_____
_____
_____
_____
_____
_____
_____
_____
_____
_____
_____
_____
_____

Typhus – Scrub

Weapon
No

Alternate Names
Miteborn typhus fever
Tsutsugamushi disease

Etiology
R. tsutsugamushi

Transmission
Source:	Mites
Entry:	Mite bite
Human-to-Human:	No

Predisposing/Comorbid Conditions
NA

Demographics
Location:	Asia, Australia
Populations:	All, esp new occupation military forces
Calendar:	Year-round

Systems
Gastrointestinal
Lymphatic
Respiratory – lower
Skin

Incubation
1-3 weeks

Signs/Symptoms
Breath sounds, gen – crackling (rales)
Chest – cough, NS
Eyes, conjunctivae – injected
Head – pain (headache)
Heart rate – slow relative to fever (relative bradycardia)
Liver – enlarged (hepatomegaly)
Lymph nodes – enlarged [1]
Lymph nodes – tender
Mentation – confusion
Mentation – delirium
Muscles – pain (myalgia)
Nausea
Skin, general – rash, macular [2]
Skin, single lesion – endurated, red (eschar) [4] [5]
Skin, single lesion – necrosis [3]
Skin, sweating – increased (hyperhidrosis)
Spleen – enlarged (splenomegaly)
Temperature, body – elevated (fever)

Differentiation
Includes, but not limited to:
Typhus – epidemic
Typhus – murine

Complications
Include, but not limited to:
Bleeding
Circulatory failure
Myocarditis
Pneumonia
Renal failure
Spontaneous abortion

Laboratory
Blood liver enzymes – increased
Blood lymphocytes – increased (lymphocytosis)
Blood platelets – decreased (thrombocytopenia)
Blood serology – positive

ECG

NA in absence of complications

Imaging

NA in absence of complications

Other Tests

NA in absence of complications

Treatment – Nonpharmacologic

NS

Treatment – Pharmacologic

Antibiotics

　　Chloramphenicol

　　Doxycycline

　　Tetracycline

Treatment – Surgical/Invasive

NA in absence of complications

Precautions

Standard

Primary Prevention

Vaccine: no

Mite control

Repellants

Course

Variable

Mortality with treatment – rare

Mortality without treatment – up to 60% ▲

Notes

[1]   Most prominent in region of primary lesion

[2]   Begins on trunk, spreads to extremities

[3]   After a few days

[4]   Multiloculated vesicle

[5]   Site of infected mite attachment

http://www.argus1.com/?tyscrub

Updates

Venezuelan Equine Encephalitis

Weapon
CDC Bioterrorism Category: B

Alternate Names
VEE
Venezuelan encephalitis
Venezuelan equine fever

Etiology
VEE virus (togaviridae, *alphavirus*)

Transmission
Source:	Rodent-mosquito cycle
Entry:	Mosquito (*culex, aedes*, others) bite
	Aerosol in laboratory
Human-to-Human:	No

Predisposing/Comorbid Conditions
NA

Demographics
Location:	South and Central America, Trinidad, SW USA
Populations:	All, esp children
Calendar:	Year-round

Systems
Nervous

Incubation
1-6 days

Signs/Symptoms [1, 2]

Chills
Consciousness – loss, prolonged (coma)
Eyes, retroorbital – pain
Head – pain (headache)
Mentation – confused
Mentation – delirium
Mentation – feeling of weakness (malaise)
Mentation – sleepiness (somnolence)
Mood – labile
Mood – lethargic
Mood – restless, irritable
Muscles – pain (myalgia)
Muscles – paralysis
Muscles – weak
Nausea
Neck, posterior – pain
Neck, posterior – stiff (meningismus)
Seizures
Signs/symptoms, nervous system – multiple other
Temperature, body – elevated (fever)
Throat – sore
Vomiting

Differentiation

Includes, but not limited to:
Other causes of encephalitis

Complications

Inappropriate ADH secretion
Neurological, i.e., personality change, paralysis (long-term)

Laboratory [3] ▲

Blood culture – positive
Blood IgG-specific antibodies – present
Blood IgM-specific antibodies – present
Blood liver enzymes – increased
Blood lymphocytes – decreased (lymphopenia)
Blood platelets – decreased (thrombocytopenia)

ECG

NA in absence of complications

Imaging

NA in absence of complications

Other Tests

NA in absence of complications

Treatment – Nonpharmacologic

Fluids, electrolytes

Treatment – Pharmacologic

NS

Treatment – Surgical/Invasive

NA

Precautions

BSL-3 procedures ▲

Primary Prevention

Vaccine: investigational
Mosquito bite protection
Mosquito control

Course

Most cases mild, self-limited, without neurological involvement, esp adults
Mortality low

Notes

[1]   Most cases have mild, self-limited course without neurologic symptoms
[2]   Sudden onset of initial non-neurologic symptoms
[3]   BSL-3 procedures ▲

http://www.argus1.com/?vee

Updates

Viral Gastroenteritis

Weapon
No

Alternate Names
Stomach flu
Stomach virus

Etiology [1]
Rotavirus, enteric adenovirus, astrovirus, caliciviruses (includes norovirus)

Selective infection of small intestine villus tip cells

Transmission
Source: Humans
Entry: Ingestion
Human-to-Human: Yes

Predisposing/Comorbid Conditions
More severe with immune deficiency, bowel disease, malnutrition

Demographics
Location: Global
Populations: All; more severe in infants
Calendar: Year-round

Systems
Gastrointestinal

Incubation
$^{1}/_{2}$–3 days depending on agent

Signs/Symptoms
Abdomen – cramps
Bowel movements – diarrhea

Bowel sounds – increased
Head – pain (headache)
Nausea
Mentation – malaise
Muscles – pain (myalgia)
Temperature, body – elevated (fever) [2]
Vomiting

Differentiation

Includes, but not limited to:
Appendicitis
Bacterial infections
Bowel obstruction
Food poisoning
Intussusception
Other causes of gastroenteritis
Protozoal infections

Complications

Include, but not limited to:
Dehydration
Necrotizing enterocolitis

Laboratory [4]

Blood arterial pH – decreased (acidosis) [3]
Blood concentration – increased [3]

ECG

NA in absence of complications

Imaging

NA in absence of complications

Other Tests

NA in absence of complications

Treatment – Nonpharmacologic

Fluids and electrolytes

Treatment – Pharmacologic

Antidiarrheals
Antiemetics

Treatment – Surgical/Invasive
NA in absence of complications

Precautions
Standard [5]

Primary Prevention
Avoidance/control of contaminated water [6]

Hygiene [5]

Course
Recovery in 1-3 days in otherwise healthy persons

Notes
[1]   Rarely determined

[2]   Often normal and low-grade when present

[3]   Caused by dehydration

[4]   Stools are negative for WBC and blood

[5]   Esp hand-washing

[6]   Esp water supply of close population groups, i.e., cruise ships for norovirus prevention

http://www.argus1.com/?viralgastro

Updates

_____

_____

_____

_____

_____

_____

_____

_____

_____

_____

_____

_____

_____

_____

Viral Rhinitis

Weapon
No

Alternate Names
Common cold
Nasopharyngitis

Etiology
Many viruses including
Adenovirus
Coxsackie
Echovirus
Influenza
Parainfluenza
Rhinovirus [4]
Respiratory syncytial virus (RSV)

Transmission
Source: Humans
Entry: Direct contact of infected secretions to mucus membrane of eyes, nose
                       Inhalation of secretions
Human-to-Human: Yes

Predisposing/Comorbid Conditions
NA

Demographic
Location: Global
Populations: All
Calendar: Seasonal, varying with virus

Systems
Oropharynx

Incubation

1-3 days

Signs/Symptoms

Breath sounds – coarse (rhonchi)
Chest, ant – pain/burning/tightness, nonpleuritic [1]
Cough – nonproductive
Cough – productive [2]
Eyes, tears (lacrimation) – increased
Head – pain (headache)
Mentation – weak (malaise)
Muscles – pain (myalgia)
Nose, drainage – increased (rhinorrhea, coryza)
Nose – congested
Nose – sneezing
Smell sense – decreased/absent (anosmia)
Taste sense – decreased/absent
Temperature, body – elevated (fever) [3]
Throat – injected
Throat – sore
Voice – hoarse

Differentiation

Includes, but not limited to:
Allergic rhinitis
Influenza
Sinusitis

Complications

Include, but not limited to:
Asthma exacerbation
Bacterial bronchitis
Bacterial sinusitis
Otitis media

Laboratory

Nose secretion culture – positive [5]

ECG

NA

Imaging
NA in absence of complications

Other Tests
NA in absence of complications

Treatment – Nonpharmacologic
Warm vapor inhalation

Treatment – Pharmacologic
Symptomatic only [6] ▲

Treatment – Surgical/Invasive
NA

Precautions
Standard

Primary Prevention
Vaccine: no
Avoid exposure
Handwashing

Course
Self-resolving in days

Notes
[1]   Due to tracheitis
[2]   Scanty sputum
[3]   Children < age 3 years, low grade if present
[4]   20-40% of cases
[5]   May identify virus in 20-35% of cases
[6]   Avoid aspirin and aspirin-containing products for febrile infections in
      children < age 19 years due to association with Reye's syndrome ▲

http://www.argus1.com/?viralrhin

Updates

_____

_____

_____

_____

_____

_____

_____

_____

_____

_____

_____

_____

_____

_____

_____

_____

_____

_____

_____

_____

West Nile Fever

Weapon
No

Alternate Names
SLEV
West Nile encephalitis [9]

Etiology
Flavavirus

Transmission

Source:	Many animals, esp birds; humans
Entry:	Mosquito bite
	Contact with infected animals?
	Blood transfusion
	Organ transplantation
	Breast feeding
Human-to-Human:	Yes

Predisposing/Comorbid Conditions
Hypertension [10]
Immune deficiency

Demographics

Location:	Global
Population:	All; risk increases with age
Calendar:	Temperate climates – late summer-early fall
	Tropics – year-round

Systems
Gastrointestinal
Lymphatic
Musculoskeletal
Nervous

Optic
Skin

Incubation
3-14 days

Signs/Symptoms [5]
Abdomen – pain
Appetite – decreased (anorexia)
Back – pain
Bowel movements – diarrhea
Chills
Consciousness – altered
Consciousness – loss, prolonged (coma)
Cough – nonproductive
Eyes, conjunctivae – injected
Eyes, light sensitivity – increased (photophobia)
Eyes, motion gen – decreased/paralyzed (ophthalmoplegia)
Eyes, retroorbital – pain
Eyes, vision – loss, subtotal
Face, muscles unilat – weak
Gait – ataxic
Extremities, hands/feet – numb
Head – pain (headache)
Joints – pain (arthralgia)
Liver – enlarged (hepatomegaly)
Lymph nodes – enlarged
Mentation – confusion
Mentation – delirium
Mentation – weak (malaise)
Mood – lethargic
Muscles, movement gen – spontaneous
Muscles, unilat – paralysis (hemiplegia) [3]
Muscles, unilat – weak (hemiparesis) [3]
Muscles – pain (myalgia)
Muscles – tremors, intention
Muscles – weak [1]
Nausea
Neck, post – stiff (meningismus)
Seizures

Sign: Kernig's
Skin – rash, red (erythematous)
Skin – rash, macular/papular
Skin – rash, roseola-like
Speech – absent/loss (aphonia/aphasia)
Spleen – enlarged (splenomegaly)
Temperature, body – elevated (fever)
Tendon reflexes, gen – asymmetric
Tendon reflexes, gen – decreased [3]
Throat – injected [2]
Throat – sore [2]
Vomiting

Differentiation

Includes, but not limited to:
Cerebrovascular diseases
Guillain-Barré syndrome
Other causes of encephalitis

Complications [7]

Include, but not limited to:
Acute flaccid paralysis [8]
Basal ganglia abnormalities
Cranial neuropathies
Hepatitis
Myocarditis
Optic neuritis
Pancreatitis
Respiratory failure

Laboratory [6] ▲

Blood IgM enzyme assay – positive
Blood lymphocytes – decreased (lymphopenia) [3]
Blood WBC – increased (leukocytosis)
CSF protein – increased
CSF WBC – increased

ECG

NA in absence of complications

Imaging

CNS, leptomeninges markings – increased (MRI) [4]
CNS, perivascular markings – increased (MRI) [4]

Other Tests

NA in absence of complications

Treatment – Nonpharmacologic

NS

Treatment – Pharmacologic

NS

Treatment – Surgical/Invasive

NA in absence of complications

Precautions

BSL-3 procedures

Primary Prevention

Vaccine: no
Mosquito control and protection
Reduce workplace risk

Course

Mortality – up to 15% in severe cases ☠

Notes

[1] Profound and common in 1999 New York outbreak
[2] Uncommon
[3] More common in West Nile than other forms of encephalitis
[4] 1/3 of cases
[5] Resembles St Louis encephalitis
[6] BSL-3 procedures ▲
[7] Neurologic changes may become permanent
[8] Resembles poliomyelitis
[9] With extension of initial systemic viral infection to central nervous system
[10] May promote virus crossing blood-brain barrier

http://www.argus1.com/?westnile

Updates

_____
_____
_____
_____
_____
_____
_____
_____
_____
_____
_____
_____
_____
_____
_____
_____
_____
_____
_____

Western Equine Encephalitis

Weapon
CDC Bioterrorism Category: B

Alternate Names
WEE

Etiology
Western equine encephalitis virus, family togaviridae, genus *Alphavirus*

Transmission
Source: Mosquitoes – *culex tarsalis*
Entry: Mosquito bite
Human-to-Human: No

Predisposing/Comorbid Conditions
NA

Demographics
Location: Western (esp California) and Central USA, Western Canada, S America
Populations: All in infected areas, esp infants and children
Calendar: Year-round, peak April-September

Systems
Nervous

Incubation
3-15 days

Signs/Symptoms [2]
Abdomen – pain

Bowel movements, control – loss of
Bowel movements – diarrhea
Chills
Consciousness – loss, prolonged (coma)
Cranial nerve VII – palsy
Dizziness (vertigo, true)
Eyes, motion general – jerky (nystagmus)
Eyes, vision – light sensitivity, increased (photophobia)
Gait – ataxic
Head – pain (headache)
Joints – pain (arthralgia)
Mentation – confused
Mentation – delirium
Mentation – feeling of weakness (malaise)
Mood – labile
Mood – lethargic
Mood – restless, irritable
Muscles, movement – fine (fasciculations)
Muscles, movement – jerks (myoclonus)
Muscles, movement – spontaneous (involuntary)
Muscles – pain (myalgia)
Muscles – paralysis [1]
Muscles – weak [1]
Nausea
Neck, posterior – pain
Neck, posterior – stiff (meningismus)
Seizures
Sign: Babinski's
Signs/symptoms, nervous system – multiple other
Speech – absent (aphonia) or loss (aphasia)
Temperature, body – elevated (fever)
Throat – sore
Urination, spontaneous control – loss of (urinary incontinence, true)
Vomiting

Differentiation
Includes, but not limited to:
Other encephalitides

Complications
Include, but not limited to:
    Mild-severe permanent neurologic damage [3]
    Respiratory failure

Laboratory
    Blood IgM-specific antibodies – present
    Blood culture – positive
    Blood WBC – increased (leukocytosis)
    CSF culture – positive
    CSF IgM-specific antibodies – present
    CSF pressure – increased
    CSF protein – increased
    CSF WBC – increased

ECG
    NA in absence of complications

Imaging
    NA in absence of complications

Other Tests
    NA in absence of complications

Treatment – Nonpharmacologic
    NS

Treatment – Pharmacologic
    NS

Treatment – Surgical/Invasive
    NA

Precautions
    Standard

Primary Prevention
    Vaccine: no
    Mosquito control

Course
<5% fatal

Notes
[1]   Sudden onset; hemiparesis with tendon reflex asymmetry and positive Babinski's sign
[2]   Many persons infected with WEE virus have no symptoms or a mild ("flu-like") course without encephalitis symptoms
[3]   Esp children (30%)

http://www.argus1.com/?wee

Updates

Yellow Fever

Weapon
CDC Bioterrorism Category: A

Alternate Names
NA

Etiology
Yellow fever virus, genus *flavavirus*

Transmission
Source:	A*edes aegypti* mosquito from
	Humans – urban form
	Monkeys – jungle/sylvan form
Entry:	Mosquito bite
Human-to-Human:	No

Predisposing/Comorbid Conditions
More serious with advanced age

Demographics
Location:	Africa, S America
Populations:	All
Calendar:	Year-round

Systems
Coagulation
Cardiovascular
Gastrointestinal
Liver/Gallbladder/Pancreas
Renal

Incubation
3-6 days

Signs/Symptoms

Abdomen, epigastrium – pain

Appetite – reduced (anorexia)

Back – pain

Bowel movements, stool – blood or black (hematochezia) (melena)

Bowel movements – constipation

Chills

Eyes, conjunctivae – injected

Eyes – bleeding

Face – flushed

Head – pain (headache)

Heart rate – slow relative to fever (relative bradycardia) [1]

Heart rhythm – irregular

Hiccups

Mentation – delirium

Mentation – weakness (malaise)

Mood – restless, irritable

Mouth, gingiva – bleeding

Mouth, mucosa – hemorrhage

Mouth – blood

Muscles – pain (myalgia)

Nausea

Nose – blood (epistaxis)

Skin, color – yellow (jaundice)

Skin – rash, petechiae

Sleep – disturbed (insomnia)

Temperature, body – elevated (fever)

Tongue, center – "furred"

Tongue – reddened [2]

Urine – absent (anuria)

Urine – decreased (oliguria)

Vomiting – blood (hematemesis)

Differentiation

Includes, but not limited to:

Hepatitis

Leptospirosis

Malaria

Other hemorrhagic fevers

Rickettsial fevers

Complications

Include, but not limited to:

Acute renal tubular necrosis

Cardiac dysrhythmias

Congestive heart failure

Disseminated intravascular coagulation (DIC)

Hyperkalemia

Liver failure

Meningoencephalitis

Metabolic acidosis

Pneumonia

Seizures

Severe hemorrhage

Laboratory [3] ▲

Blood bilirubin – increased

Blood factor VII – decreased

Blood fibrinogen – decreased

Blood glucose – decreased

Blood liver enzymes – increased

Blood prothrombin time – increased

Blood PTT – increased

Blood WBC – decreased (leukopenia)

Urine protein – present (proteinuria)

ECG

Dysrhythmias, NS

PR interval – long (AV conduction – 1st degree block)

QT interval – long

Rate – slow (sinus bradycardia)

Rate – slow relative to temperature (relative bradycardia)

ST-T waves – abnormal, NS

Imaging

NA in absence of complications

Other Tests

Isolate yellow fever virus from blood

Isolate yellow fever virus from liver biopsy

Treatment – Nonpharmacologic
NS

Treatment – Pharmacologic
NS
Aspirin contraindicated ▲

Treatment – Surgical/Invasive
NA in absence of complications

Precautions
BSL-3 procedures ▲
Handling blood samples in acute phase ▲

Primary Prevention
Vaccine: yes
Place patients under net to prevent mosquito transfer to others

Course
Mortality 10-12% ☠

Notes
[1]   "Faget" sign
[2]   Esp margins
[3]   BSL-3 procedures ▲

http://www.argus1.com/?yellow

Updates

_____
_____
_____
_____
_____
_____
_____
_____
_____
_____
_____

Yersiniosis

Weapon
CDC Bioterrorism Category: B

Alternate Names
Extraintestinal yersiniosis
Intestinal yersiniosis

Etiology
Y enterocolitica

Transmission
Source: Animals, esp swine
Entry: Ingestion of contaminated food, esp under-
cooked pork, unpasteurized milk, water
Blood transfusion
Human-to-Human: No

Predisposing/Comorbid Conditions
More severe in immune deficiency

Demographics
Location: Global
Populations: All, esp children
Calendar: Year-round, peak winter

Systems
Gastrointestinal

Incubation
3-7 days

Signs/Symptoms
Abdomen – pain [3]
Abdomen, RLQ – pain [4]

Bowel movements – blood or black (hematochezia) (melena)
Bowel movements – diarrhea
Nausea
Temperature, body – elevated (fever)
Vomiting

Differentiation

Includes, but not limited to:
Appendicitis
Other causes of enterocolitis

Complications

Include, but not limited to:
Arthritis [2]
Bowel perforation (ileum)
Dehydration
Endocarditis
Erythema nodosum
Lower gastrointestinal hemorrhage
Mesenteric adenitis
Myocarditis
Organ abscess
Pharyngitis
Septicemia [1]
Tonsillitis

Laboratory

Bile culture – positive
Blood culture – positive
Blood serology – positive
Joint fluid culture – positive
Lymph node biopsy culture – positive
Stool culture – positive
Throat culture – positive
Urine culture – positive

ECG

NA in absence of complications

Imaging

NA in absence of complications

Other Tests
NA in absence of complications

Treatment – Nonpharmacologic
Fluids and electrolytes

Treatment – Pharmacologic
Antibiotics [5]
        Aminoglyclosides
        Doxycycline
        Fluroquinolones
        Trimethoprim sulfa

Treatment – Surgical/Invasive
NA in absence of complications

Precautions
Standard

Primary Prevention
Vaccine: no
Avoid contaminated products
Food handling and preparation

Course
Complete resolution usual

Notes
[1]   Esp in immune deficiency, advanced age, iron-overload states
[2]   Esp common in Scandinavia; occurs about 1 week after onset of intestinal symptoms
[3]   Due to mesenteric adenitis
[4]   May resemble acute appendicitis
[5]   Treatment of uncertain value in mild cases

http://www.argus1.com/?yers

Updates

CLINICAL GUIDE—POISONS

Ammonia Poisoning

Weapon
CDC hazardous chemical category: choking/lung/pulmonary agent

Alternate Names
NA

Etiology
Anhydrous ammonia

Converted to ammonium hydroxide aerosol when mixed with water in mucous membranes (eyes, oral mucosa, airways), causing thermal and chemical liquefaction tissue necrosis

Transmission
Source:	Industrial
Entry:	Contact
	Inhalation
	Ingestion
Human-to-Human:	No [8]

Predisposing/Comorbid Conditions
NA

Demographics
Location:	Global
Populations:	All
Calendar:	Year-round

Systems
Optic
Oropharynx
Respiratory – upper
Skin

Time to Clinical Onset
Minutes

Signs/Symptoms

Abdomen – pain
Breath sounds – coarse (rhonchi)
Breath sounds – crackling (rales)
Breath sounds – wheezes
Breathing – diff, acute (acute dyspnea)
Chest – burning
Chest – pain
Chest – tightness
Cough – acute
Cough – productive [1]
Eyes, conjunctivae – swelling (edema)
Eyes, cornea – ulcer
Eyes, tearing – excess (lacrimation)
Eyes, vision – loss [2]
Eyes, vision – blurred
Eyes – irritation
Eyes – pain
Eyes – swollen
Head – pain (headache)
Heart, rate – rapid (tachycardia)
Lips – swollen [3]
Mood – irritable
Mood – restless
Mouth – burning
Mouth – swelling [3]
Nausea
Skin – blisters [4]
Skin color – red (erythema) [4]
Skin – pain [4]
Sputum – blood (hemoptysis)
Sweating – increased (hyperhydrosis)
Temperature, body – elevated (fever)
Voice – hoarse
Vomiting

Differentiation

Includes, but not limited to:
Asthma
Other causes of acute dyspnea

Complications

Include, but not limited to:
    Bronchiectasis
    Cataracts
    Cornea perforation
    Gastrointestinal bleeding [5]
    Gastrointestinal perforation [5]
    Gastrointestinal strictures [5]
    Noncardiac pulmonary edema [6]
    Pneumonia
    Vascular collapse

Laboratory

    Blood arterial pH – decreased (acidosis)
    Blood arterial pO_2 – decreased (hypoxia)
    Blood arterial pCO_2 – increased
    Blood liver enzymes – increased

ECG

    NA in absence of complications

Imaging

    Lungs – NS [7]

Other Tests

    Bronchoscopy

Treatment – Nonpharmacologic

    Do not induce emesis ▲
    Drink water or milk for ingested poison
    Fluids
    Intubation and ventilation
    Oxygen
    Remove all clothing
    Skin/eye washing and irrigation

Treatment – Pharmacologic

    Antidote: no
    Antibiotics – ophthalmic
    Bronchodilators
    Corticosteroids (?)

Treatment – Surgical/Invasive
Bronchoscopy
Endoscopy for ingestion

Precautions
Protective clothing:	yes
Site decontamination:	yes
Other:	NS

Primary Prevention
Industrial safety

Course
Variable with exposure

Notes
[1] Copius tracheal secretions
[2] Blindness can be temporary or permanent depending on exposure
[3] May be severe
[4] Esp moist areas
[5] When ingested
[6] Due to damage of alveolocapillary membrane
[7] Consolidation and other signs of pneumonia
[8] Unless victim skin/clothing contaminated with liquid form

http://www.argus1.com/?ammonia

Updates

_____
_____
_____
_____
_____
_____
_____
_____
_____
_____
_____
_____
_____
_____

Arsenic Poisoning

Category
CDC hazardous chemical category: metal

Alternate Names
NA

Etiology
Trivalent and pentavalent arsenic compounds

Inhibition of sulfhydril cellular enzymes with damage to GI tract walls and peripheral blood vessels

Transmission
Source:	Industrial metallurgy, semiconductors, pesticides, wine, glue contamination
Entry:	Ingestion
	Inhalation (rare)
Human-to-Human:	No

Predisposing/Comorbid Conditions
NA

Demographics
Location:	Global
Populations:	All
Calendar:	Year-round

Systems
Cardiovascular
Gastrointestinal

Time to Clinical Onset
Minutes – hours

Signs/Symptoms
Abdomen – pain
Arterial press – low [1]

Bowel movements – diarrhea
Breath, odor – garlic
Eyes, vision – dim
Eyes, vision – light sensitivity, increased (photophobia)
Mouth – pain/burning
Muscles – twitching
Nausea
Seizures
Throat – burning
Voice – hoarse
Vomiting
Vomiting – blood (hematemesis)

Differentiation
Includes, but not limited to:
Other causes of acute gastroenteritis

Complications
Include, but not limited to:
Bone marrow suppression
Cardiac dysrhythmias
Coma
Dermatitis
Dehydration
Encephalopathy
Hepatic dysfunction
Intestinal perforation
Intrauterine fetal death ☠
Polyneuropathy
Renal failure
Respiratory failure

Laboratory
Urine arsenic – increased

ECG
Dysrhythmias

Imaging
Intestinal arsenic on plain radiography [2]

Other Tests
Cardiac monitoring for dysrhythmias

Treatment – Nonpharmacologic
Fluids and electrolytes
Hemodialysis
Skin/eye washing and irrigation
Ventilation
Whole-bowel irrigation

Treatment – Pharmacologic
Antidote: no
Chelation
     dimercaprol
     D-penicillamine
     DMSA
     DMPS

Treatment – Surgical/Invasive
NA

Precautions
NA

Primary Prevention
Vaccine: no
Industrial safety

Course
Variable with exposure intensity and time to treatment

Notes
[1]   Due to volume depletion from vascular damage
[2]   Arsenic is radiopaque

http://www.argus1.com/?arsenic

Updates

Arsine Poisoning

Weapon
CDC hazardous chemical category: blood agent

Alternate Names
NA

Etiology
Arsine

Depletes RBC glutathione, causing cell membrane instability and hemolysis

Transmission
Source:	Semiconductor industry
Entry:	Contact with liquid
	Inhalation [7]
Human-to-Human:	No

Predisposing/Comorbid Conditions
NA

Demographics
Location:	Global
Population:	All, esp workers exposed to metal refining, lead plating, soldering
Calendar:	Year-round

Systems
Cardiovascular
Gastrointestinal
Hematopoietic/Immune [2]
Renal/Genitourinary
Skin

Time to Clinical Onset
Minutes – hours [6]

Signs/Symptoms [5] ▲
Abdomen, flank – pain
Abdomen – pain
Arterial press – low
Breath, odor – garlic
Breathing – difficult (dyspnea)
Breathing – rapid (tachypnea)
Dizziness (lightheaded)
Eyes, conjunctivae – red stain
Head – pain (headache)
Heart rate – rapid (tachycardia)
Heart sound – S3 LV [5]
Liver – enlarged (hepatomegaly)
Mentation – disorientation
Mentation – memory loss
Mentation – restless, agitated
Mentation – weakness (malaise)
Muscles – cramps
Muscles – pain (myalgia)
Muscles – weak
Nausea
Skin color – bronze
Skin – freezing [7]
Thirst – excessive
Urine – blood (hematuria)
Vomiting

Differentiation
Includes, but not limited to:
Other causes of congestive heart failure
Other causes of hemolytic anemia

Complications
Include, but not limited to:
Congestive heart failure
Dehydration
Encephalopathy/encephalitis
Hyperkalemia
Myocarditis
Noncardiac pulmonary edema
Peripheral neuropathy
Renal failure

Laboratory

Blood BNP – increased [5]
Blood calcium – decreased
Blood CPK – increased
Blood haptoglobin – present
Blood Hgb/Hct – decreased (anemia)
Blood liver enzymes – increased
Blood myoglobin – present
Blood potassium – increased
Blood RBC – fragments
Blood WBC – decreased (leukopenia)
Urine hemoglobin – positive [1]
Urine protein – present (proteinuria)

ECG [5]

Abnormalities – nonspecific
Rate – rapid (sinus tachycardia)
ST segment – depressed [3]
T wave – peaked [4]

Imaging

NS

Other Tests

NA in absence of complications

Treatment – Nonpharmacologic [8]

Fluids and electrolytes
Hemodialysis
Transfusion
Urine alkalinization
Ventilation with oxygen

Treatment – Pharmacologic

Antidote: no
Chelation therapy (?)

Treatment – Surgical/Invasive

NA in absence of complications

Precautions

Protective clothing: yes
Site decontamination: yes
Other: SCBA

Primary Prevention

Industrial safety

Course

Variable with exposure [6]

Notes

[1]   + for blood but no RBC's on microscopic exam
[2]   Acute hemolytic anemia due to depletion of erythrocyte glutathione, causing RBC membrane instability
[3]   Due to myocardial ischemia
[4]   Due to hyperkalemia
[5]   Although the heart is not primarily involved in arsine poisoning, cardiac failure may quickly occur and may predominate by the time patients are first seen ▲
[6]   Death may occur within 30 minutes ☠
[7]   Frostbite
[8]   For skin contact with liquid, gentle removal of clothing and skin washing

http://www.argus1.com/?arsine

Updates

_____
_____
_____
_____
_____
_____
_____
_____
_____
_____
_____
_____
_____

Barium Poisoning

Category
CDC hazardous chemical category: metal

Alternate Names
NA

Etiology
Soluble barium [1]

Proposed mechanism of toxicity is blockage of cellular efflux of potassium, but not uptake, causing hypokalemia, which may be severe

Transmission
Source: Industrial
Entry: Ingestion
Human-to-Human: No

Predisposing/Comorbid Conditions
NA

Demographics
Location: Global
Populations: All
Calendar: Year-round

Systems
Cardiovascular
Gastrointestinal
Musculoskeletal

Time to Clinical Onset
Minutes

Signs/Symptoms

Abdomen, epigastrium – pain
Bowel movements – diarrhea
Heart, rhythm – irregular [2]
Heart rate – slow (bradycardia)
Muscles – paralysis [2, 3]
Muscles – weak [2, 3]
Nausea
Tendon reflexes – reduced or absent [2]
Vomiting

Differentiation [4]

Includes, but not limited to:
Tetrodotoxin poisoning
Tick paralysis
Other causes of paralysis

Complications

Include, but not limited to:
Renal failure
Rhabdomyolysis
Ventricular fibrillation

Laboratory

Blood aldolase – increased
Blood creatine phosphokinase (CPK) – increased
Blood creatinine – increased
Blood phosphate – decreased
Blood potassium – decreased
Blood urea nitrogen – increased

ECG

AV conduction – AV dissociation, complete
Dysrhythmias, ventricular
QRS – long
Rate – slow (sinus bradycardia)
U wave – prominent

Imaging
NA in absence of complications

Other Tests
NA in absence of complications

Treatment – Nonpharmacologic
Fluids, electrolytes – esp potassium [5] ▲
Gastric lavage
Hemodialysis
Ventilation

Treatment – Pharmacologic
Antidote: no
NS

Treatment – Surgical/Invasive
NA

Precautions
NA

Primary Prevention
Industrial safety

Course
Variable with intensity of poisoning and treatment

Notes
[1]   Include barium carbonate, barium chloride, etc; does *not* include form
      of barium used in contrast imaging, which is not absorbed
[2]   Due to hypokalemia
[3]   All extremities; lasts hours-days
[4]   Differentiated by normal potassium levels
[5]   Monitor potassium carefully to avoid hyperkalemia because total body
      potassium is normal ▲

http://www.argus1.com/?barium

Updates

Benzene Poisoning

Weapon
CDC hazardous chemical category: organic solvent

Alternate Names
Benzol
Coal tar naptha
Cyclohexatriene
Phenyl hydride

Etiology
Benzene (C_6H_6)

Irritation of exposed tissue; bone marrow suppression

Transmission
Source:	Industrial, motor fuels, paint removers
Entry:	Contact
	Ingestion
	Inhalation
Human-to-Human:	No

Predisposing/Comorbid Conditions
NA

Demographic
NA

Systems
Cardiovascular
Gastrointestinal
Hematopoietic
Nervous
Optic
Skin

Time to Clinical Onset
Immediate

Signs/Symptoms
Abdomen – pain
Appetite – decreased
Bowel movements – diarrhea
Breathing, rate – increased (tachypnea)
Chest – tightness
Consciousness – loss, prolonged (coma) [2]
Consciousness – loss, sudden (syncope) [2]
Dizziness (lightheaded)
Extremities – tremors
Eyes, conjunctivae – injected
Eyes, vision – blurred
Eyes – irritation
Gait – unsteady
Head – pain (headache)
Heart rate – rapid (tachycardia)
Heart rhythm – irregular [3]
Mentation – confused
Mentation – sleepy (somnolence)
Mentation – weakness (malaise)
Mood – depressed [1]
Mood – euphoric [1]
Muscles – tremors
Nausea
Seizures
Skin – blisters
Skin color – red (erythema)
Skin – pain
Vomiting

Differentiation
Includes, but not limited to:
Other dermatologic, gastrointestinal, mucosal irritants

Complications
Include, but not limited to:
Aspiration pneumonitis
Bone marrow suppression

Cardiac dysrhythmias
Coma
Cornea injury
Leukemia
Noncardiac pulmonary edema
Renal Failure
Respiratory failure

Laboratory

Blood Hgb/Hct – decreased (anemia)
Blood liver enzymes – increased
Blood platelets – decreased (thrombocytopenia)
Blood WBC – decreased (leukopenia)
Urine phenol – increased

ECG

Dysrhythmias

Imaging

Pulmonary edema

Other Tests

NS in absence of complications

Treatment – Nonpharmacologic

Do not induce emesis ▲
Fluids and electrolytes
Gastric lavage
Oxygen
Skin/eye washing and irrigation
Ventilation

Treatment – Pharmacologic

Antidote: no
Caution using sympathomimetics [3] ▲
NS

Treatment – Surgical/Invasive

NA in absence of complications

Precautions

Protective clothing: yes
Site decontamination: yes
Other: SCBA

Primary Prevention
Industrial safety

Course
Variable with exposure intensity

Notes
[1] Initial euphoria or excitement followed by depression
[2] Consciousness usually returns after removed from exposure, but may have prolonged coma
[3] May precipitate cardiac dysrhythmias, esp ventricular fibrillation, due to increased myocardial sensitivity to circulating catecholamines

http://www.argus1.com/?benzene

Updates

_____
_____
_____
_____
_____
_____
_____
_____
_____
_____
_____
_____
_____
_____
_____
_____
_____
_____
_____
_____
_____
_____
_____

Brevetoxin Poisoning

Weapon
CDC hazardous chemical category: biotoxin

Alternate Names
Neurotoxic shellfish poisoning
NSP
Red tide toxin

Etiology
Brevetoxin [3]

Blocks action potentials in nerves by preventing sodium flow, reducing nerve conduction

Transmission
Source: Shellfish
Entry: Ingestion
                     Inhalation
Human-to-Human: No

Predisposing/Comorbid Conditions
NA

Demographics
Location: Coasts – global
Populations: All
Calendar: Year-round, sporadic

Systems
Gastrointestinal
Nervous
Respiratory – upper [1]

Time to Clinical Onset

Ingestion: <1 hour-18 hours
Inhalation: immediate

Signs/Symptoms

Abdomen – pain
Bowel movements – diarrhea
Breathing – diff, acute (acute dyspnea) [1]
Breath sounds – wheezes [1]
Cough – acute NS [1]
Dizziness (true vertigo)
Extremities – pain, shooting (paresthesias)
Gait – ataxic
Sensation, hot and cold temperature – reversed
Vomiting

Differentiation

Includes, but not limited to:
Asthma [1]
Gastroenteritis – all causes
Menniere's disease

Complications

Include, but not limited to:
Dehydration

Laboratory

Blood, ELISA antibodies – positive [2]

ECG

NA in absence of complications

Imaging

NA in absence of complications

Other Tests

NA in absence of complications

Treatment – Nonpharmacologic

NS

Treatment – Pharmacologic
Antidote: no
NS

Treatment – Surgical/Invasive
NA

Precautions
NA

Primary Prevention
NS

Course
Self-limited with complete recovery

Notes
[1]   Inhaled form
[2]   Not certified for detection
[3]   Lipophilic polyether neurotoxin produced by red tide dinoflagellate *gymnodinium breve*

http://www.args1.com/?breve

Updates

_____
_____
_____
_____
_____
_____
_____
_____
_____
_____
_____
_____
_____
_____

Bromine Poisoning

Weapon
CDC hazardous chemical category: choking/lung/pulmonary agent

Alternate Names
NA

Etiology
Bromine gas (Br_2)

Irritation of exposed tissue

Transmission
Source:	Industrial, i.e., gasoline additive, agriculture, sanitation, fire retardant
Entry:	Contact with liquid/gas
	Ingestion of contaminated food/water
	Inhalation of gas
Human-to-Human:	No

Predisposing/Comorbid Conditions
NA

Demographics
Location:	Global
Populations:	All, esp chemical plant workers
Calendar:	Year-round

Systems
Gastrointestinal
Optic
Oropharynx
Respiratory – lower
Respiratory – upper
Skin

Time to Clinical Onset
Minutes

Signs/Symptoms
Abdomen – pain
Breathing – diff, acute (acute dyspnea)
Breathing – rapid (tachypnea)
Cough – acute NS
Cough – productive
Dizziness (lightheaded)
Eyes, conjunctivae – injected
Eyes, vision – light sensitivity, increased (photophobia)
Eyes – tearing, excess (lacrimation)
Head – pain (headache)
Mentation – weakness (malaise)
Mouth, mucosa color – brown
Mouth – burning
Nausea
Nose – blood (epistaxis)
Nose – irritation
Skin – brown discoloration
Skin – irritation
Skin – itching (pruritus)
Skin – rash, pustular
Skin – rash, vesicular
Sweating – increased (hyperhydrosis)
Tongue – brown discoloration
Vomiting

Differentiation
Includes, but not limited to:
Chlorine poisoning

Complications
Include, but not limited to:
Hemorrhagic gastroenteritis
Noncardiac pulmonary edema
Pneumonitis
Skin ulcers

ECG
NS in absence of complications

Laboratory
Blood bromide – increased

Imaging
NS in absence of complications

Other Tests
NS in absence of complications

Treatment – Nonpharmacologic
Skin/eye washing and irrigation
Ventilation

Treatment – Pharmacologic
Antidote: no
NS

Treatment – Surgical/Invasive
NA in absence of complications

Precautions
Protective clothing: yes
Site decontamination: yes
Other: NS

Primary Prevention
Industrial safety

Course
Variable with exposure

http://www.argus1.com/?bromine

Updates

_____

_____

_____

_____

_____

_____

_____

_____

_____

_____

_____

_____

_____

_____

_____

_____

_____

_____

_____

_____

_____

_____

_____

BZ Poisoning

Weapon
CDC hazardous chemical category: incapacitating agent

Alternate Names
Agent 15

Etiology
3-quinuclidinyl benzilate

Inhibition of acetylcholine in autonomic and central nervous
systems

Transmission
Source:	Military weapon
Entry:	Contact
	Ingestion
	Inhalation
Human-to-Human:	No

Predisposing/Comorbid Conditions
NA

Demographics
Location:	Global
Populations:	All
Calendar:	Year-round

Systems
Nervous

Time to Clinical Onset
$^1/_2$-48 hours

Signs/Symptoms

Abdomen – pain
Arterial press – elevated
Arterial press – upright, low (orthostatic hypotension)
Behavior – bizarre or changed
Behavior – hyperactive
Bladder, urinary – distended
Bowel movements – constipation
Bowel sounds – decreased/absent (ileus, adynamic)
Consciousness – altered [2]
Consciousness – loss, prolonged (coma)
Dizziness (lightheaded)
Eyes, pupils – dilated (mydriasis)
Eyes, vision – blurred
Face – flushed
Heart rate – rapid (tachycardia) [1]
Heart rate – slow (bradycardia) [1]
Mentation – concentration impaired
Mentation – confabulation
Mentation – confused
Mentation – crying, purposeless
Mentation – disrobing
Mentation – hallucinations
Mentation – illusions
Mentation – judgement impaired
Mentation – memory impaired (amnesia)
Mentation – paranoid
Mentation – smiling/laughter, inappropriate
Mood – anxious
Mood – combative
Mood – fearful
Mood – labile
Mood – restless, irritable
Mouth – dry (xerostomia)
Muscles – movement, incoordinated (ataxia)
Muscles – weak
Skin – dry
Skin – flushed
Skin – temperature, hot
Speech – inarticulate (dysarthria)

Sweating – decreased
Temperature, body – elevated (fever)
Tendon reflexes – increased (hyperactive reflexes)
Thirst – excessive
Urination force – decreased
Vomiting

Differentiation

Includes, but not limited to:
Alcohol intoxication
Anxiety reaction
Hallucinogenic substances, i.e., LSD
Other causes of anticholinergic syndrome
Schizophrenia and other CNS mood and mental disorders

Complications

Include, but not limited to:
Cardiac dysrhythmias
Dehydration
Electrolyte disturbances
Hyperthermia-induced
Self-inflicted injury

Laboratory

Urine BZ – present

ECG

NA in absence of complications

Imaging

NA in absence of complications

Other Tests

NA in absence of complications

Treatment – Nonpharmacologic

Decontamination of clothing
Fluids and electrolytes
Isolation from hazardous objects
Skin washing

Treatment – Pharmacologic
Antidote: physostigmine

Treatment – Surgical/Invasive
NA

Precautions
Protective clothing: yes
Site decontamination: yes
Other: NA

Primary Prevention
NS

Course
Variable with exposure intensity and time to treatment

Notes
[1]   Tachycardia initially
[2]   BZ-induced hallucinations become realistic and decrease in size with time

http://www.argus1.com/?bz

Updates

_____
_____
_____
_____
_____
_____
_____
_____
_____
_____
_____
_____
_____
_____
_____

Carbon Monoxide Poisoning

Weapon
CDC hazardous chemical category: blood agent

Alternate Names
NA

Etiology
Carbon monoxide (CO)

Fixation of CO to hemoglobin (Hgb) increases binding of O_2 to Hgb and reduces release of O_2 to peripheral body tissues [1]

Transmission
Source:	Many, including propane engines, auto exhaust, natural gas appliances, fireplaces, grills, paint, generators
Entry:	Inhalation
Human-to-Human:	No

Predisposing/Comorbid Condition
NA

Demographics
Location:	Global
Populations:	All
Calendar:	Year-round, peak winter

Systems
Cardiovascular
Coagulation [2]
Gastrointestinal [2]

Musculoskeletal [2]
Nervous
Optic
Respiratory – lower [2]
Skin

Time to Clinical Onset
Minutes [9]

Signs/Symptoms
Abdomen – pain
Arterial press – low
Behavior – bizarre or changed
Bowel movements, control – loss
Bowel movements, stool – blood or black (hematochezia) (melena)
Bowel movements – diarrhea
Breathing – diff, rest (rest dyspnea)
Breathing – rapid (tachypnea)
Breath sounds – crackling (rales)
Chest, ant – pain, nonpleuritic rest
Chest, ant – palpitations
Consciousness – altered
Consciousness – loss, prolonged (coma)
Consciousness – loss, sudden (syncope)
Dizziness (lightheaded)
Ears, hearing – loss (deafness)
Ears – ringing (tinnitus)
Eyes, motion – jerky (nystagmus)
Eyes, retina – hemorrhage, flame-shaped
Eyes, retina – papilledema
Eyes, retroorbital – pain
Eyes, vision – blurred
Eyes, vision – loss, subtotal
Eyes, vision – scotoma
Gait – ataxic
Hair – loss (alopecia)
Head, gen – pain (headache)
Heart rate – rapid (tachycardia)
Heart rhythm – irregular

Mentation – concentration impaired
Mentation – confused
Mentation – judgement impaired
Mentation – memory impaired (amnesia)
Mentation – NS changes
Mentation – sleepiness (somnolence)
Mentation – weakness (malaise)
Mood – anxious
Mood – depressed
Mood – lethargic
Muscles – rigid
Muscles – tremors, rest
Muscles – weak
Nausea
Seizures
Skin color – cherry red
Skin color – erythematous patches
Sputum – blood (hemoptysis)
Urination spontaneous control – loss (urinary incontinence, true)
Vomiting

Differentiation

Includes, but not limited to:
Alcohol intoxication
Cerebrovascular accident
Congestive heart failure
Food poisoning
Primary neuropsychiatric conditions

Complications

Include, but not limited to:
Acute myocardial infarction [7] ▲
Blindness
Diabetes insipidus
Disseminated intravascular coagulation
Dysrhythmias
Lactic acidosis
Noncardiac pulmonary edema
Rhabdomyolysis
Thrombotic thrombocytopenic purpura

ECG
Dysrhythmias, ventricular [6] ▲
Rate – rapid (sinus tachycardia)
ST-T wave – NS abnormality [3]

Laboratory
Blood amylase – increased [4]
Blood arterial pH – decreased (acidosis)
Blood calcium – decreased
Blood carboxyhemoglobin – increased [5]
Blood glucose – increased

Imaging
NA in absence of complications

Other Tests
NA in absence of complications

Treatment – Nonpharmacologic
Oxygen – 100% [8] ▲

Treatment – Pharmacologic
Antidote: oxygen ▲

Treatment – Surgical/Invasive
NA in absence of complications

Precautions
Protective clothing: No
Site decontamination: Ventilation
Other: SCBA

Primary Prevention
Household/industrial precautions [10]

Course
Variable with exposure intensity and prior health, esp cardiac and
CNS conditions
Recovery may take weeks

Notes

[1]   "Haldane effect"; brain and heart, which are esp O_2-dependent for metabolism, are most severely affected

[2]   Involvement indicates severe poisoning

[3]   May be due to myocardial ischemia

[4]   Salivary gland origin

[5]   Correlates poorly with clinical severity

[6]   Lowered threshold for ventricular fibrillation, even at carboxyhemoglobin levels <10% ▲

[7]   Esp patients with prior coronary heart disease ▲

[8]   Administer at greater than atmospheric pressure (hyperbaric oxygenation)

[9]   Immediate "intoxication" syndrome; may be followed days later by recurrence of symptoms

[10]   Carbon monoxide detector, esp near gas-burning appliances

http://www.argus1.com/?carmox

Updates

_____
_____
_____
_____
_____
_____
_____
_____
_____
_____
_____
_____
_____
_____
_____
_____
_____
_____
_____
_____
_____
_____

Chlorine Poisoning

Weapon

CDC hazardous chemical category: choking/lung/pulmonary agent

Alternate Names

NA

Etiology

Chlorine gas

Toxic effects due to formation of hydrochlorous and hydrochloric acid when comes into contact with water in body tissue, causing tissue necrosis and coagulation defects

Transmission

Source:	Industrial, water purifiers, disinfectants
Entry:	Inhalation
Human-to-Human:	No

Predisposing/Comorbid Conditions

NA

Demographics

Location:	Global
Populations:	All
Calendar:	Year-round

Systems

Coagulation
Optic
Oropharynx
Respiratory – lower
Skin

Time to Clinical Onset
Immediate

Signs/Symptoms
Abdomen – pain
Arterial pressure – increased [7]
Arterial pressure – decreased [7]
Breath sounds, local – wheezes
Breath sounds – coarse (rhonchi)
Breath sounds – crackling (rales)
Breathing – difficult, acute (dyspnea)
Breathing – rapid (tachypnea)
Chest, ant – pain/tightness, nonpleuritic
Chest – cough, acute NS
Chest – rales
Chills
Consciousness – altered
Consciousness – loss, sudden (syncope)
Dizziness (lightheaded)
Eyes, conjunctivae – injected
Eyes, cornea – burns
Eyes, tearing (lacrimation) – increased
Eyes – irritation
Head – pain (headache)
Heart rate – rapid (tachycardia)
Mentation – weakness (malaise)
Mood – anxious
Mouth – burning
Nausea
Nose – irritation
Skin, face – burns [6]
Skin color – blue (cyanosis)
Skin – pain [6]
Sputum – blood (hemoptysis)
Temperature, body – elevated (fever) [1]
Temperature, body – decreased (hypothermia) [1]
Throat – injected
Throat – sore
Voice – hoarse
Vomiting

Differentiation

Includes, but not limited to:
    Asthma
    Congestive heart failure
    Other causes of acute cough with or without dyspnea
    Other causes of acute pulmonary edema
    Pulmonary embolus

Complications

Include, but not limited to:
    Noncardiac pulmonary edema
    Respiratory failure
    Respiratory infection

Laboratory

    Blood arterial pH – decreased [3]
    Blood arterial pH – increased [2]
    Blood arterial pO_2 – decreased (hypoxia)
    Blood WBC – increased (leukocytosis)

Imaging

    Lungs, parenchyma – consolidation [4]
    Lungs, parenchyma interstitial markings – increased
    Lungs, vasculature – congested [5]

Other Tests

    NA in absence of complications

Treatment – Nonpharmacologic

    Oxygen
    Skin/eye washing and irrigation

Treatment – Pharmacologic

    Bronchodilators
    Corticosteroids
    Nonsteroidal anti-inflammatory drugs (?)

Treatment – Surgical/Invasive

    NA

Precautions

Protective clothing:	yes
Site decontamination:	yes
Other:	SBCA

Primary Prevention

Industrial safety

Course

Variable with intensity and duration of exposure
Full recovery usual

Notes

[1]   Mild
[2]   Respiratory alkalosis
[3]   Metabolic acidosis
[4]   Focal areas of consolidation
[5]   Central congestion
[6]   Exposed areas, esp face
[7]   Initially increased, then decreased

http://www.argus1.com/?chlorine

Updates

_____
_____
_____
_____
_____
_____
_____
_____
_____
_____
_____
_____
_____
_____
_____
_____
_____
_____
_____
_____

Colchicine Poisoning

Weapon
CDC hazardous chemical category: biotoxin

Alternate Names
NA

Etiology
Extract of *colchicum autumnale*

Toxic effect caused by binding to tubulin, inhibiting cell mitosis

Transmission
Source:	Medicine
	Saffron leaves [1]
Entry:	Ingestion
	Intravenous
Human-to-Human:	No

Predisposing/Comorbid Conditions
Major depression with suicide intention

Demographics
Location:	Global
Populations:	All
Calendar:	Year-round

Systems
Cardiovascular
Coagulation
Gastrointestinal
Hematopoietic/Immune
Musculoskeletal
Nervous
Renal/Genitourinary
Respiratory – lower

Time to Clinical Onset
4-12 hours

Signs/Symptoms [3]
Abdomen – pain
Appetite – decreased
Bowel movements, stool – blood or black (hematochezia) (melena)
Bowel movements – diarrhea
Liver – enlarged (hepatomegaly)
Mentation – coma
Mentation – delirium
Seizures
Skin, hair – loss (alopecia) [4]
Vomiting
Vomiting – blood (hematemesis)

Differentiation
Includes, but not limited to:
All causes of acute gastroenteritis
All other causes of multi-organ failure
Arsenic poisoning
Nonsteroidal anti-inflammatory drug poisoning
Other medical poisons

Complications
Include, but not limited to:
Acute renal failure
Acute respiratory failure
Cardiac dysrhythmias
Dehydration
Disseminated intravascular coagulation
Electrolyte abnormalities
Neutropenia
Rhabdomyolysis
Seizures
Sepsis
Shock
Thrombocytopenia

Laboratory [3]
Blood WBC – increased (leukocytosis)
Blood WBC – left shift [2]
Liver enzymes – increased
Urine protein – present
Urine RBC – present

ECG
Dysrhythmias

Imaging
NA in absence of complications

Other Tests
NA in absence of complications

Treatment – Nonpharmacologic
Fluids and electrolytes
Gastric lavage

Treatment – Pharmacologic
Antidote: no
NS

Treatment – Surgical/Invasive
NA

Precautions
NA

Primary Prevention
Home medicinal safety

Course
Variable with exposure and time-to-treatment

Notes
[1]   May be mistaken for leaves of ransom herb *allium ursinum*
[2]   May include immature myeloid cells

[3]   Not including findings of multi-organ failure beginning 24-72 hours after acute exposure involving systems listed

[4]   Late occurrence

http://www.argus1.com/?colchicine

Updates

_____

_____

_____

_____

_____

_____

_____

_____

_____

_____

_____

_____

_____

_____

_____

_____

_____

Cyanide Poisoning

Weapon
CDC hazardous chemical category: blood agent

Alternate Names
Cassava poisoning
Konzo

Etiology [5]
Cyanogen chloride
Hydrogen cyanide
Potassium cyanide
Sodium cyanide

Toxic effects caused by cyanide binding of ferric iron in mitochondrial cytochrome oxidase, affecting cellular ability to utilize O_2 in oxidative phosphorylation, causing tissue hypoxia, anaerobic metabolism and lactic acidosis

Transmission
Source:	Industrial, fires, poisonous plants [7]
Entry:	Inhalation
	Ingestion
Human-to-Human:	No

Predisposing/Comorbid Condition
NA

Demographics
Location:	Global
Populations:	All, esp chemical industry workers
Calendar:	Year-round

Systems
Cardiovascular
Hematopoietic/Immune

Nervous
Optic
Respiratory – lower
Respiratory – upper
Rhabdomyolysis

Time to Clinical Onset

Immediate

Signs/Symptoms [3]

Abdomen, epigastrium – pain
Arterial press – elevated
Arterial press – low
Bowel movements – diarrhea
Breath, odor – "bitter almonds" or musty
Breathing – deep (hyperpnea)
Breathing – diff, rest (rest dyspnea)
Breathing – rapid (tachypnea)
Chest, ant – pain, nonpleuritic rest
Chest, ant – palpitations
Chest – rales
Consciousness – loss, prolonged (coma)
Consciousness – loss, sudden (syncope)
Cough – acute, NS
Dizziness (lightheaded)
Eyes, conjunctivae – injected
Eyes, pupil reaction – slow
Eyes, pupils – dilated (mydriasis)
Eyes, tearing (lacrimation) – increased
Eyes – pain
Head – pain (headache)
Heart rate – rapid (tachycardia)
Heart rate – slow (bradycardia)
Heart rhythm – irregular
Mentation – coma
Mentation – sleepy (somnolence)
Mentation – syncope
Mood – anxious
Mood – restless/irritable
Nausea
Nose – drainage (rhinorrhea, coryza)

Seizures
Skin color – blue (cyanosis) [1]
Skin – pain
Throat – sore
Vomiting

Differentiation
Includes, but not limited to:
All other causes of acute respiratory failure

Complications
Include, but not limited to:
Noncardiac pulmonary edema [4]
Respiratory failure
Seizures
Shock

Laboratory
Blood lactate – increased [6]
Blood pH – decreased

ECG [2] ▲
AV conduction – 1st degree block
AV conduction – 2nd degree block, Mobitz II
AV conduction – 3rd degree block
Dysrhythmias, atrial
Dysrhythmias, ventricular
Rate – rapid (sinus tachycardia)
Rate – slow (sinus bradycardia)
ST segment – depressed
T wave – inversion, abnormal

Imaging
Chest x-ray – NS in absence of complications

Other Tests
NS in absence of complications

Treatment – Nonpharmacologic
Do not induce vomiting for ingestion ▲

Eye/skin irrigation and washing
Rest
Ventilation with oxygen

Treatment – Pharmacologic
Antidote: no
NS

Treatment – Surgical/Invasive
NA in absence of complications

Precautions
Protective clothing: yes
Site decontamination: yes
Other: SBCA
Do not administer mouth-to-mouth artificial respiration ▲
Wear protective gloves when administering first aid ▲
Avoid any skin-skin contact with victims ▲
No food or liqiud ingestion or smoking during care ▲
Remove contaminated clothes following aid ▲

Primary Prevention
Industrial safety

Course
Varies with exposure intensity
Less than 5% overall mortality

Notes
[1]   Late only; skin color typically normal or cherry red in presence of hypoxia
[2]   Cardiac rhythm should be continuously monitored ▲
[3]   Depend on route, dose of exposure, i.e., inhalation vs gastrointestinal
[4]   Both inhalation and gastrointestinal exposure
[5]   Compounds that release cyanide spontaneously, by thermal decomposition, or by chemical reaction, such as cyanogen, cyanogen bromide, cyanogen chloride, calcium cyanide, acetonitrile, laetrile, amygdalin, lethane, thanate, sodium nitroprusside, cassava root

[6]   Usually normal

[7]   Smoke inhalation: combined carbon monoxide and cyanide poisoning

http://www.argus1.com/?cyanide

Updates

Digitalis Poisoning

Category
CDC hazardous chemical category: biotoxin

Alternate Names
Digitalis intoxication [1]

Etiology
Digitalis medicinal preparations
>> Taken in excess [2]
>> Increased sensitivity

Decreases intracardiac impulse conduction and suppresses/stimulates cardiac impulse generation

Transmission
Source: Medicine
Entry: Ingestion
                     Parenteral
Human-to-Human: No

Predisposing/Comorbid Conditions
Advanced age
Cardiac disease
Drugs
>> amiodarone
>> corticosteroids
>> cylclosporine
>> diuretics
>> other cardiac drugs
Electrolyte abnormalities
Endocrine/metabolic disease
Kidney disease
Pulmonary disease

Demographics
Location: Global
Populations: All, esp aged
Calendar: Year-round

Systems
Cardiovascular
Gastrointestinal
Nervous

Time to Clinical Onset
Variable

Signs/Symptoms
Abdomen – pain
Appetite – reduced (anorexia)
Bowel movements – diarrhea
Chest, ant – palpitations
Consciousness – loss, sudden (syncope)
Dizziness (lightheaded)
Eyes, vision – blurred
Eyes, vision – colored halos around lights
Face – pain
Fatigue
Heart rate – slow (bradycardia)
Heart rate – rapid (tachycardia)
Heart rhythm – irregular
Mentation – confused
Mentation – weakness (malaise)
Mood – depressed
Nausea
Sleep – disturbed (insomnia)
Urination – nocturnal (nocturia)
Vomiting

Differentiation
Includes, but not limited to:
CNS and mood disorders, esp major depression
Gastroenteritis
Other causes of cardiac dysrhythmias

Complications

Include, but not limited to:
Advanced atrioventricular heart block
Cardiac ventricular fibrillation

Laboratory

Blood digitalis level – increased [3]
Blood potassium – decreased

ECG

Dysrhythmias, atrial
Dysrhythmias, conduction block
Dysrhythmias, junctional
Dysrhythmias, ventricular
Rate – slow (sinus bradycardia)
ST segment – depressed
ST-T wave – abnormality, NS
Tachycardia – bidirectional

Imaging

NA in absence of complications

Other Tests

NA

Treatment – Nonpharmacologic

DC digitalis
DC drugs that elevate digitalis blood levels
Fluids and electrolytes
Oxygen for hypoxia

Treatment – Pharmacologic

Digoxin-specific antibodies [6]
Potassium [4] ▲
Lidocaine [5]
Phenytoin [5]

Treatment – Surgical/Invasive

Dialysis
Ventricular pacing

Precautions

NA

Primary Prevention

Careful monitoring of medical status, esp potassium, of patients taking digitalis

Course

Variable depending on concurrent conditions and level of intoxication

Notes

[1]   Also called digitalis glycoside, digitoxin, digoxin

[2]   Small separation between therapeutic and toxic effects, making toxic levels easily achieved in patients taking drugs in this class

[3]   Interpret only in the context of other factors, esp low blood potassium and hypoxia, which increase sensitivity to digitalis

[4]   Contraindicated if heart block or hyperkalemia is present ▲

[5]   For ventricular dysrhythmias

[6]   Digiband

http://www.argus1.com/?digitalis

Updates

_____
_____
_____
_____
_____
_____
_____
_____
_____
_____
_____
_____
_____
_____

Elemental Mercury Poisoning—Acute

Category
CDC hazardous chemical category: metal

Alternate Names
Quicksilver
Hydragyrum
Metal fume fever

Etiology
Elemental mercury (Hg^{0+})

Binds to sulfide groups, blocking sulfhydril enzymes, disrupting cellular metabolism

Transmission
Source:	Industrial, medicinal
Entry:	Inhalation [1]
	Ingestion [2]
Human-to-Human:	No

Predisposing/Comorbid Condition
NA

Demographics
Location:	Global
Populations:	All
Calendar:	Year-round

Systems
Nervous
Respiratory – upper
Respiratory – lower

Time to Clinical Onset
Minutes-hours

Signs/Symptoms [3]
Arterial pressure – increased
Bowel movements – diarrhea
Breathing – diff, acute (acute dyspnea)
Chest – pain
Chills
Cough, non-productive
Eyes – irritation
Heart rate – increased (tachycardia)
Mentation – coma
Mentation – confusion
Mentation – weakness (malaise)
Mood – lethargic
Mouth, gingiva – inflamed
Mouth – burning
Nausea
Sense of taste – metallic
Skin – rash, erythematous
Skin – rash, vesicular
Vomiting

Differentiation
Includes, but not limited to:
Other causes of acute respiratory distress

Complications [3]
Include, but not limited to:
Chronic mercury poisoning
Noncardiac pulmonary edema
Respiratory failure

Laboratory
Blood mercury – increased
Urine mercury – increased

ECG
NA in absence of complications

Imaging
NA in absence of complications

Other Tests
NA in absence of complications

Treatment – Nonpharmacologic [3]
Skin/eye washing and irrigation
Ventilation with humidified oxygen

Treatment – Pharmacologic [3]
Antidote: no
Chelation therapy if systemic absorption occurs

Treatment – Surgical/Invasive
NA

Precautions
Protective clothing:	yes
Site decontamination:	yes
Other:	NS

Primary Prevention
Home safety
Industrial safety

Course
Variable with exposure intensity
Chronic poisoning may occur with systemic absorption

Notes
[1]   Easily vaporizes from liquid form at room temperature to become inhaled and converted in vivo to inorganic form, which is toxic to respiratory tract

[2]   Important mainly in persons with abnormal GI absorption as elemental mercury is otherwise poorly absorbed

[3]   Acute inhaled form only

http://www.argus1.com/?mercury

Updates

_____

_____

_____

_____

_____

_____

_____

_____

_____

_____

_____

_____

_____

_____

_____

_____

_____

_____

_____

Ethylene Glycol Poisoning

Weapon
CDC hazardous chemical category: toxic alcohol

Alternate Names
1,2-dihydroxyethane
1,2-ethanediol
2-hydroxyethanol
Ethylene alcohol
Ethylene dihydrate
Glycol

Etiology
Ethylene glycol ($C_2H_6O_2$)

Toxic effects due to breakdown products causing metabolic acidosis and formation of calcium oxalate crystals in kidneys and other tissues

Transmission
Source:	Industrial, i.e., antifreeze, de-icing solutions, and polyester fibers; ingredient in hydraulic brake fluids and in various inks; solvent in paints and plastics
Entry:	Ingestion
Human-to-Human:	No

Predisposing/Comorbid Condition
Alcoholism

Demographics
Location:	Global
Populations:	All, esp persons working with cars and photographic developing solutions
Calendar:	Year-round

Systems
Nervous
Renal/Genitourinary

Exposure to Clinical Onset
Hours [3]

Signs/Symptoms [1, 5]
Arterial press – elevated
Arterial press – low
Consciousness – loss, prolonged (coma)
Consciousness – loss, sudden (syncope)
Dizziness (lightheaded)
Eyes, motion – jerky (nystagmus)
Eyes, motion – reduced or paralyzed (ophthalmoplegia)
Gait – unsteady (ataxia)
Head – pain (headache)
Heart rate – rapid (tachycardia)
Mentation – confusion [1]
Mentation – sleepy (somnolence)
Mood – restless/irritable
Muscles – spasm (myoclonus) [4]
Nausea
Seizures
Speech – slurred
Tendon reflexes – reduced or absent
Vomiting
Vomiting – blood (hematemesis)

Differentiation
Includes, but not limited to:
Ethyl alcohol intoxication

Complications
Include, but not limited to:
Cerebral edema
Congestive heart failure
Hypocalcemia
Hyperkalemia
Metabolic acidosis

Neuropathy
Noncardiac pulmonary edema
Renal failure – oliguric
Respiratory failure
Shock

Laboratory
Blood – anion gap
Blood arterial pH – decreased (acidosis)
Blood calcium – increased
Blood potassium – increased

ECG
Dysrhythmias – NS [2]

Imaging
NS in absence of complications

Other Tests
NS in absence of complications

Treatment – Nonpharmacologic
Gastric lavage
Hemodialysis

Treatment – Pharmacologic
Sodium bicarbonate [6]

Treatment – Surgical/Invasive
NA in absence of complications

Precautions
NA

Primary Prevention
Industrial safety

Course
Untreated: variable, sometimes fatal ☠

Notes

[1] Appear "drunk" but without alcohol on breath
[2] Due to hyperkalemia
[3] Varies with exposure intensity
[4] Due to hypocalcemia
[5] First 24 hours, after which signs of renal failure may occur
[6] Correction of metabolic acidosis

http://www.argus1.com/?ethylene

Updates

_____
_____
_____
_____
_____
_____
_____
_____
_____
_____
_____
_____
_____
_____
_____
_____
_____
_____
_____
_____
_____

Lewisite Poisoning

Weapon
CDC hazardous chemical category: blister agent/vessicant

Alternate Names
"L"

Etiology
Lewisite

Causes direct cell damage, mechanism unknown

Transmission
Source:	Military weapon
Entry:	Contact
	Ingestion of contaminated food/water
	Inhalation
Human-to-Human:	No

Predisposing/Comorbid Conditions
NA

Demographics
Location:	Global
Populations:	All
Calendar:	Year-round

Systems
Optic
Respiratory – upper
Skin

Time to Clinical Onset
Immediate

Signs/Symptoms
Abdomen – pain
Arterial press – low [1]
Bowel movements – blood (melena)
Bowel movements – diarrhea
Breathing – diff, acute (acute dyspnea)
Breath sounds – wheezes
Chest – pain, burning
Cough – productive [3]
Eyes, conjunctivae – edema
Eyes, conjunctivae – injected
Eyes, cornea – damage
Eyes, lids – (edema) swelling
Eyes, vision – light sensitivity, increased (photophobia)
Eyes, vision – loss, binocular total (blindness)
Eyes, vision – loss, transient (temporary blindness)
Eyes – blinking, spasmodic (blepharospasm)
Eyes – pain
Eyes – tearing, excess
Head, sinuses – pain
Mentation – weakness (malaise)
Mood – restless, irritable
Nausea
Nose – blood (epistaxis)
Nose – drainage (rhinorrhea, coryza)
Nose – irritation
Nose – sneezing [2]
Skin, local – blisters
Skin color – gray [4]
Skin color – red (erythematous)
Temperature, body – decreased (hypothermia)
Voice – hoarse
Vomiting

Differentiation
Includes, but not limited to:
Other dessicants and blistering agents

Complications
Include, but not limited to:
Bone marrow suppression

Hepatic failure
Noncardiac pulmonary edema
Renal failure

Laboratory
NA in absence of complications

ECG
NA in absence of complications

Imaging
NA in absence of complications

Other Tests
NA in absence of complications

Treatment – Nonpharmacologic
Do not induce emesis ▲
Eye/skin irrigation and washing
Rapid decontamination
Ventilation

Treatment – Pharmacologic
Antidote: British anti-lewisite

Treatment – Surgical/Invasive
NA

Precautions
Protective clothing: yes
Site decontamination: yes
Other: SCBA

Primary Prevention
NA

Course
Variable with exposure intensity

Notes

[1] "Lewisite shock" due to hypovolemia
[2] May be violent
[3] Frothy sputum
[4] Sign of tissue death that may appear minutes after exposure

http://www.argus1.com/?lewisite

Updates

_____

_____

_____

_____

_____

_____

_____

_____

_____

_____

_____

_____

_____

_____

_____

_____

_____

_____

_____

_____

Methyl Bromide Poisoning

Weapon

CDC hazardous chemical category: choking/lung/pulmonary agent

Alternate Names

Bromomethane
Embafume
Isobrone
Monobromomethane
Methyl fume
Terabol

Etiology

Methyl bromide (CH_3Br)

Methylation of sulfhydryl groups, disrupting cell function, esp CNS

Transmission

Source:	Natural – from oceanic algae and kelp
	Industrial – fumigant, sod preparation [1]
Entry:	Contact
	Inhalation
Human-to-Human:	No

Predisposing/Comorbid Condition

NA

Demographics

Location:	Global
Populations:	All
Calendar:	Year-round

Systems

Nervous

Optic
Respiratory – upper
Skin

Time to Clinical Onset
1-48 hours

Signs/Symptoms
Breathing – diff, rest (rest dyspnea)
Chest – pain
Consciousness – loss, prolonged (coma)
Cough – acute NS
Dizziness (lightheaded)
Eyes, movements – involuntary
Eyes, pupils – dilated
Eyes, vision – blurred
Eyes, vision – double (diplopia)
Eyes – irritation
Eyes – tearing, excess (lacrimation)
Gait – ataxic
Head – pain (headache)
Mentation – delirium
Mentation – manic
Mentation – weakness (malaise)
Mood – anxious
Mood – euphoric
Mood – restless, irritable
Nausea
Seizures
Skin color – erythema
Skin – itching (pruritus)
Skin – pain
Skin – rash, vesicular
Speech – inarticulate (dysarthria)
Tendon reflexes – decreased
Throat – irritation
Touch sensation – decreased
Vomiting

Differentiation

Includes, but not limited to:

    Other causes of CNS abnormailites

    Other inhalational and blistering agents

Complications

Include, but not limited to:

    Blindness

    Brain damage

    Corneal injury

    Hepatic failure

    Neuropsychosis

    Noncardiac pulmonary edema

    Optic nerve atrophy

    Peripheral neuropathy

    Pneumonitis

    Respiratory failure

    Renal failure

Laboratory

    Blood arterial pO_2 – decreased (hypoxia)

    Blood liver enzymes – increased

    Blood urea nitrgen – increased

Imaging

    NA in absence of complications

Other Tests

    Pulse oximetry

Treatment – Nonpharmacologic

    Eye/skin irrigation and washing

    Remove and discard clothing

    Ventilation with oxygen

Treatment – Pharmacologic

    Antidote: no

    Activated charcoal (ingestion)

    Bronchodilators

Treatment – Surgical/Invasive
NA

Precautions
Protective clothing: yes
Site decontamination: yes
Other: NA

Primary Prevention
Industrial safety

Course
Variable with intensity of exposure

Note
[1]   Highly destructive to ozone layer; industrial uses being phased out

http://www.argus1.com/?methylbromide

Updates

_____
_____
_____
_____
_____
_____
_____
_____
_____
_____
_____
_____
_____
_____
_____
_____
_____
_____
_____
_____

Methyl Isocyanate Poisoning

Weapon
CDC hazardous chemical category: choking/lung/pulmonary agent

Alternate Names
Isocyanatomethane
Methyl carbylamine
MIC

Etiology
Methyl isocyanate (C_2H_3NO)

Irritation/corrosion of respiratory tract

Transmission
Source:	Industrial, i.e., pesticides, rubber, adhesives
Entry:	Contact
	Inhalation
Human-to-Human:	No

Predisposing/Comorbid Condition
NA

Demographics
Location:	Global
Populations:	All
Calendar:	Year-round

Systems
Optic
Respiratory – lower
Respiratory – upper
Skin

Time to Clinical Onset
1-4 hours

Signs/Symptoms
Abdomen – pain
Bowels – defecation
Breathing – diff, acute (acute dyspnea)
Breathing – rapid (tachypnea)
Breath sounds – wheezes
Breath sounds – crackling (rales)
Chest, ant – pain, nonpleuritic rest
Consciousness – loss, sudden (syncope)
Cough – acute nonspecific
Eyes, conjunctivae – injected
Eyes, cornea – damage
Eyes, lids – swelling (edema)
Eyes, light sensitivity – inceased (photophobia)
Eyes – irritation
Eyes – tearing, excess (lacrimation) [1]
Mouth – burning
Nausea
Nose – irritation
Skin – burns
Vomiting

Differentiation
Includes, but not limited to:
Asthma

Complications
Include, but not limited to:
Eye damage
Noncardiac pulmonary edema
Pneumonia
Respiratory failure

Laboratory
NA in absence of complications

ECG

NA in absence of complications

Imaging

NA in absence of complications

Other Tests

NS in absence of complications

Treatment – Nonpharmacologic

Eye/skin irrigation and washing
Fluids/electrolytes
Remove contaminated clothing
Ventilation

Treatment – Pharmacologic

Antidote: no
Bronchodilators
Corticosteroids

Treatment – Surgical/Invasive

NA

Precautions

Protective clothing: yes
Site decontamination: yes
Other: SCBA

Primary Prevention

Industrial safety

Course

Variable and may be fatal ☠

Note

[1]   Highly sensitive indicator of exposure

http://www.argus1.com/?methyliso

Updates

_____

_____

_____

_____

_____

_____

_____

_____

_____

_____

_____

_____

_____

_____

_____

Nicotine Poisoning

Weapon
CDC hazardous chemical category: biotoxin

Alternate Names
NA

Etiology
Nicotine

Stimulation, followed by suppression, of nicotinic
cholinergic ganglia

Transmission
Source:	Tobacco leaves, commercial tobacco, nicotine patch, nicotine gum, insecticides
Entry:	Ingestion
Human-to-Human:	No

Predisposing/Comorbid Conditions
NA

Demographics
Location:	Global
Populations:	All, esp children
Calendar:	Year-round

Systems
Cardiovascular
Nervous

Time to Clinical Onset
Hours

Signs/Symptoms
Abdomen – pain
Arterial press – elevated
Arterial press – low [1]
Bowel movements – diarrhea
Breathing – diff, acute (acute dyspnea)
Breathing – rapid (tachypnea)
Chest, ant – palpitations
Consciousness – loss, prolonged (coma)
Consciousness – loss, sudden (syncope)
Head – pain (headache)
Heart rate – rapid (tachycardia)
Heart rate – slow (bradycardia) [1]
Mentation – confused
Mentation – weakness (malaise)
Mood – depressed
Mood – restless, irritable
Mouth – burning
Mouth – drooling
Nausea
Seizures
Skin color – pale (palor)
Sputum – excessive (bronchorrhea)
Sweating – increased
Vomiting

Differentiation
Includes, but not limited to:
Organophosphate poisoning

Complications
Include, but not limited to:
Respiratory failure
Shock

Laboratory
NS in absence of complications

ECG

NS in absence of complications

Imaging

NA in absence of complications

Other Tests

NA in absence of complications

Treatment – Nonpharmacologic

Gastric irrigation
Skin irrigation
Ventilation

Treatment – Pharmacologic

Antidote: atropine
Activated charcoal (ingestion)

Treatment – Surgical/Invasive

NA

Precautions

NA

Primary Prevention

Home medicinal/tobacco exposure precautions

Course

Variable with exposure intensity

Note

[1]   Severe exposure

http://www.argus1.com/?nicotine

Updates

_____

_____

_____

_____

_____

_____

_____

_____

_____

_____

_____

_____

_____

_____

_____

_____

_____

_____

_____

_____

Opioid Poisoning

Weapon
CDC hazardous chemical category: incapacitating agent

Alternate Names
NA

Etiology
Codeine
Fentanyl
Heroin
Meperidine
Methadone
Morphine
Propoxyphene

Inhibit synaptic transmission via stimulation of
opioid receptors in central and peripheral nervous system

Transmission
Source: Legal and illicit substances
Entry: Ingestion
                   Inhalation
                   Innoculation
Human-to-Human: No

Predisposing/Comorbid Conditions
Alcoholism
Drug addiction
Major depression with suicidal intent

Demographics
Location: Global
Populations: All
Calendar: Year-round

Systems
Nervous
Respiratory – lower

Time to Clinical Onset
Varies with transmission route

Signs/Symptoms
Breathing – cessation [2]
Breathing – diff, rest (rest dyspnea) [1]
Breathing – rapid (tachypnea) [1]
Breathing – slow [2]
Breath sounds – crackling (rales) [1]
Consciousness – loss, prolonged (coma)
Eyes, pupils – constricted (miosis)
Mentation – sleepiness (somnolence)
Mood – depressed
Mood – lethargic

Differentiation
Includes, but not limited to:
Congestive heart failure
Other causes of central nervous system depression

Complications
Include, but not limited to:
Cardiac conduction disturbances and dysrhythmias
Myocardial ischemia
Noncardiac pulmonary edema [1]
Seizures

Laboratory
Drug screens

ECG
NS in absence of complications

Imaging
Pulmonary edema without cardiac enlargement [1]

Other Tests
NS in absence of complications

Treatment – Nonpharmacologic
Gastric lavage (ingestion)
Ventilation with oxygen ▲

Treatment – Pharmacologic
Antidotes: opioid antagonists
     nalmefene
     naloxone
     naltrexone
Activated charcoal (ingestion)
Induce emesis (ingestion)

Treatment – Surgical/Invasive
NA

Precautions
NA

Primary Prevention
Avoidance

Course
Variable with exposure intensity, time to treatment, prior health
of victim, other substances taken, and other factors

Notes
[1]   Noncardiogenic pulmonary edema is most often due to heroin intoxication and may occur within minutes
[2]   Hypoxia due to respiratory depression is most common cause of
death ☠

http://www.argus1.com/?opioid

Updates

_____

_____

_____

_____

_____

_____

_____

_____

_____

_____

_____

_____

_____

_____

_____

_____

_____

_____

_____

_____

Organophosphate Poisoning

Poison
CDC hazardous chemical category: nerve agent

Alternate Names
Insecticide poisoning
Nerve agents

Etiology
Commercial insecticides
GF
Sarin
Soman
Tabun
VX

Cholinesterase inhibition causing widespread neurologic effects, esp muscle and CNS function

Transmission
Source: Weapon arsenals; commercial compounds
Entry: Contact
                   Ingestion
                   Inhalation
Human-to-Human: No

Demographics
Location: Global
Populations: All
Calendar: Year-round

Systems
Gastrointestinal
Nervous

Optic
Respiratory – lower

Time to Clinical Onset
Immediate

Signs/Symptoms [6]
Abdomen – pain
Arterial press – elevated
Arterial press – low (hypotension)
Bowel movements, control – loss [1]
Bowel movements – diarrhea
Breathing – cessation [1]
Breathing – diff, rest (rest dyspnea)
Breathing – rapid (tachypnea)
Chest – pain/tightness
Chest – rales
Consciousness – loss, prolonged (coma) [1]
Consciousness – loss, sudden (syncope) [1]
Cough – acute NS
Eyes, conjunctivae – injected [2]
Eyes, pupils – constricted (miosis)
Eyes, tearing (lacrimation) – increased [2]
Eyes, vision – blurred
Eyes, vision – dim
Eyes – pain [2]
Gait – unsteady [1]
Head – pain (headache)
Heart rate – increased (tachycardia)
Heart rate – decreased (bradycardia)
Mentation, memory – impaired (amnesia) [5]
Mentation, judgement – impaired [5]
Mentation – confusion [5]
Mentation – sleepy (somnolence) [5]
Mentation – weak (malaise) [5]
Mood – anxious [5]
Mood – restless/irritable [5]
Mood – depressed [5]
Mouth – drooling
Muscles, movements local – fasciculations

Muscles – paralysis [3]
Muscles – weak
Nausea
Nose, drainage – increased (rhinorrhea, coryza)
Nose – congested
Salivation – excessive (psyalism)
Seizures [1]
Skin, local – sweating [4]
Speech – slurred
Sweating – increased (hyperhydrosis)
Throat – pain/tightness
Urination, spontaneous control – decreased/absent (urinary incontinence)
Urination – frequent (polyuria)
Vomiting

Differentiation
Includes, but not limited to:
All nerve agent (organophosphate) poisonings

Complications
Include, but not limited to:
Coma
Pancreatitis
Paralysis
Respiratory failure

Laboratory
Blood arterial pH – increased
Blood cholinesterase – decreased
Blood creatine kinase (CK) – increased
Blood amylase – increased
Blood glucose – increased
Blood WBC – increased (leukocytosis)

ECG
Dyrhythmias – slow-rate (bradyarrhythmias)
Rate – decreased (sinus bradycardia)
Rate – increased (sinus tachycardia)

Imaging
NA in absence of complications

Other Tests
NA in absence of complications

Treatment – Nonpharmacologic
Airway
Do not induce vomiting for ingestion ▲
Gastric lavage
Oxygen
Remove all clothing immediately ▲
Wash entire skin immediately ▲

Treatment – Pharmacologic
Antidotes: atropine ▲
    atropine
    pralidoxime chloride
Activated charcoal

Treatment – Surgical/Invasive
NA in absence of complications

Precautions
Protective clothing: yes
Site decontamination: yes
Other: NS

Primary Prevention
Industrial safety

Course
Recovery usual with mild or moderate exposure
Survival usual with prompt treatment
Usually fatal with severe exposure ☠

Notes
[1]   Severe poisoning
[2]   Local eye symptoms have rapid onset after exposure (seconds to minutes)
[3]   Flaccid

[4]   Area of contact

[5]   CNS manifestations may persist for several weeks after acute effects end

[6]   Highly variable according to agent, causing frequent misdiagnosis

http://www.argusl.com/?organ

Updates

_____
_____
_____
_____
_____
_____
_____
_____
_____
_____
_____
_____
_____
_____
_____
_____
_____
_____

Osmium Tetroxide Poisoning

Weapon

CDC hazardous chemical category: choking/lung/pulmonary agent

Alternate Names

Osmic acid anhydride
Osmium oxide

Etiology

Osmium tetroxide (OsO_4)

Toxic effect by direct tissue oxidation

Transmission

Source:	Industrial, biology laboratories
Entry:	Contact
	Ingestion
	Inhalation
Human-to-Human:	No

Predisposing/Comorbid Conditions

NA

Demographics

Location:	Global
Populations:	All
Calendar:	Year-round

Systems

Gastrointestinal
Optic
Respiratory – lower
Respiratory – upper
Skin

Time to Clinical Onset
Hours ▲

Signs/Symptoms
Abdomen – pain (ingestion)
Breathing – diff, acute (acute dyspnea)
Breathing – rapid (tachypnea)
Breath sounds – crackling (rales)
Breath sounds – wheezes
Cough – acute NS
Dizziness (lightheaded)
Eyes, conjunctivae – injected
Eyes, cornea – black
Eyes, cornea – damage
Eyes, vision – blurred
Eyes, vision – loss, binocular total (blindness)
Eyes, vision – loss, subtotal
Eyes – irritation
Eyes – tearing, excess (lacrimation)
Head – pain (headache)
Nose – irritation
Skin color – black
Skin – irritation
Skin – pain, burning
Skin – rash, erythematous
Skin – rash, vesicular
Throat – pain
Vomiting

Differentiation
Includes, but not limited to:
Phosgene poisoning
Sarin poisoning
Sulfur mustard poisoning

Complications
Include, but not limited to:
Corneal injury/blindness
Noncardiac pulmonary edema
Pneumonia

Laboratory

NS in absence of complications

ECG

NS in absence of complications

Imaging

NS in absence of complications

Other Tests

NS in absence of complications

Treatment – Nonpharmacologic

Remove contaminated clothing
Skin/eye washing and irrigation ▲
Ventilation

Treatment – Pharmacologic

Antidote: no

Treatment – Surgical/Invasive

NA

Precautions

Protective clothing: yes
Site decontamination: yes
Other: NS

Primary Prevention

Industrial precautions

Course

Variable with exposure
May be fatal due to pulmonary damage ☠

http://www.argus1.com/?osmium

Updates

_____

_____

_____

_____

_____

_____

_____

_____

_____

_____

_____

_____

_____

_____

_____

_____

_____

_____

_____

_____

_____

Phosgene Poisoning

Poison
CDC hazardous chemical category: blister agent/vessicant

Alternate names
Carbonic acid dichloride
Carbonic dichloride
Carbon oxychloride
Carbonyl chloride
Chemical ID: ID1076
Chlorofornyl chloride

Etiology
Phosgene ($COCl_2$)

Hydrolyzes in mucous membrane water to form hydrochloric acid, damaging respiratory tract epithelial cells and eyes and also causing hemoconcentration, hypovolemia, hypoxia, liver necrosis, pulmonary necrosis, and renal necrosis

Transmission
Source:	Industrial; many household solvents, cleaning fluids, paint removers; welding in confined space
Entry:	Contact
	Inhalation
Human-to-Human:	No

Predisposing/Comorbid Conditions
NA

Demographics
Location:	Global
Populations:	All, esp chemical plant workers
Calendar:	Year-round

Systems
Optic
Oropharynx
Respiratory – upper
Skin

Time to Clinical Onset
Immediate

Signs/Symptoms [1]
Breathing – diff, acute (acute dyspnea)
Breathing – rapid (tachypnea)
Breath sounds – wheezes
Chest, ant – pain, nonpleuritic rest
Chest, ant – pain, pleuritic
Cough – acute NS
Eyes, conjunctivae – injected
Eyes, cornea – damage
Eyes, tearing (lacrimation) – increased
Eyes – irritation
Head – pain (headache)
Nausea
Nose, mucosa – inflamed
Nose – irritation
Skin color – blue (cyanosis)
Skin – irritation [2]
Sputum – blood (hemoptysis)
Sputum – clear/thick
Thirst – increased
Throat – injected
Throat – burning
Throat – dry
Vomiting

Differentiation
Includes, but not limited to:
Acute respiratory distress syndrome
Ammonia poisoning
Chlorine poisoning
Congestive heart failure

Nitrogen oxide poisoning
Pneumonia
Sulfur dioxide poisoning
Upper respiratory tract infections

Complications
Include, but not limited to:
Hemolytic anemia
Hepatic necrosis
Noncardiac pulmonary edema
Renal necrosis
Respiratory distress
Shock

Laboratory
Blood arterial pO_2 – decreased (hypoxia)
Blood bilirubin – increased
Blood concentration – increased
Blood creatinine – increased
Blood Hgb/Hct – decreased (anemia)
Blood liver enzymes – increased
Blood lung enzymes – increased
Blood urea nitrogen – increased

ECG
NS in absence of complications

Imaging
Lungs, hila bilateral – enlarged
Lungs, parenchyma central – infiltrates
Lungs, vasculature – congested

Other Tests
NS in absence of complications

Treatment – Nonpharmacologic
Oxygen
Skin/eye washing and irrigation
Ventilation

Treatment – Pharmacologic

Antidote: no
Bronchodilators
Corticosteroids
Prophylactic antibiotics

Treatment – Surgical/Invasive

NA in absence of complications

Precautions

Protective clothing:	yes
Site decontamination:	yes
Other:	SCBA

Primary Prevention

Industrial safety

Course

Untreated, varies with intensity and duration of exposure
May be fatal ☠

Notes

[1]   Initial symptoms may be followed by latent asymptomatic period of minutes after intense exposure and up to 3 days after mild exposure, followed by return of s/s

[2]   May resemble frostbite

http://www.argus1.com/?phosgene

Updates

_____
_____
_____
_____
_____
_____
_____
_____
_____
_____
_____
_____

Phosphine Poisoning

Weapon
CDC hazardous chemical category: choking/lung/pulmonary agent

Alternate Names
Chemical ID: 2199
Aluminum phosphide (AlP)
Calcium phosphide
Hydrogen phosphide
PH3
Phosphorous trihydride
Zinc phosphide (ZnP)

Etiology
Phosphine gas (PH_3) [7]

Inhalation of gas (rare) or ingestion of solid phosphide reacts with gastric HCl to form phosphine gas, which interferes with enzymes and protein synthesis, primarily in mitochondria of heart and lung cells, causing myofibril necrosis and secondary ionic changes in peripheral small vessels and lungs

Transmission
Source:	Industrial, i.e., semi-conductors, metal pickling, manufacture of phosphonium halides; contaminant of aceylene
Entry:	Inhalation
	Ingestion
Human-to-Human:	No

Predisposing/Comorbid Conditions
Major depression [8]

Demographics

Location:	Global
Populations:	All
Calendar:	Year-round

Systems

Cardiovascular
Gastrointestinal
Liver/Biliary tract/Pancreas
Nervous
Respiratory – lower

Exposure to Clinical Onset

Hours [9]

Signs/Symptoms [9]

Abdomen – pain
Arterial press, gen – decreased (hypotension) [1]
Bowel movements – diarrhea
Bowel sounds – decreased/absent (ileus, adynamic)
Breathing – difficult, acute (acute dyspnea)
Breathing – rapid (tachypnea)
Breath sounds – crackles (rales)
Chest – pain/tightness
Consciousness – loss, prolonged (coma)
Cough – acute NS
Dizziness (lightheaded)
Extremities, sensation – decreased
Extremities, sensation – "shooting" pain (paresthesia)
Eyes, vision – double (diplopia)
Gait – unsteady
Head – pain (headache)
Heart rate – increased (tachycardia)
Heart rhythm – irregular
Liver – large (hepatomegaly)
Mentation – lightheaded
Mood – restless/irritable
Muscles – tremors, intention
Nausea
Seizures [2]
Skin color – yellow (jaundice)

Spleen – enlarged (splenomegaly)
Tendon reflexes – reduced/absent
Urine volume – decreased (oliguria)
Urine – blood (hematuria)
Vomiting

Differentiation
Includes, but not limited to:
Congestive heart failure
Coronary heart disease
Primary myocardial disease

Complications
Include, but not limited to:
Hepatic failure
Noncardiac pulmonary edema
Renal failure
Shock

Laboratory
Blood arterial pH – decreased (acidosis) [4]
Blood bilirubin – increased
Blood cardiac enzymes – increased
Blood creatinine – increased
Blood Hgb/Hct – decreased (anemia)
Blood liver enzymes – increased
Blood magnesium – increased [3]
Blood urea nitrogen – increased
Blood WBC – decreased (leukopenia)
Urine protein – present (proteinuria)
Urine – blood

ECG [5, 6]
Atrium – infarction
AV conduction – AV dissociation, complete
Dysrhythmias, atrial
Dysrhythmias 2° to conduction block
QRS – RBBB pattern

Rate, general – rapid
ST segment – depressed
ST segment – elevated
T wave – inversion, abnormal

Imaging

Lungs, parenchyma – edema

Other Tests

NS in absence of complications

Treatment – Nonpharmacologic

Fluids
Gastric lavage with permanganate for ingestion ▲
Oxygen
Remove all contaminated clothing
Skin/eye washing and irrigation

Treatment – Pharmacologic

Antidote: no
Antiarrhythmics
Calcium gluconate and 20% magnesium sulfate
Restore plasma volume
Sodium bicarbonate

Treatment – Surgical/Invasive

NA in absence of complications

Precautions

Protective clothing: no
Site decontamination: yes
Other: SCBA

Primary Prevention

Industrial safety, esp ventilation of sites where used

Course

Varies with exposure and intervention
May be fatal ☠

Notes

[1]   Direct effect on peripheral vasculature, responds poorly to vasopressors
[2]   Severe exposure
[3]   Associated with large amount of myocardial damage
[4]   Combined respiratory and metabolic
[5]   Serious ECG abnormalities present in over 50%
[6]   ECG normalizes in a few weeks if patient survives first 24 hours
[7]   Colorless gas with rotten fish or garlic odor
[8]   Suicide attempts
[9]   Pulmonary symptoms may not occur until 72 hours after exposure

http://www.argus1.com/?phosphine

Updates

_____
_____
_____
_____
_____
_____
_____
_____
_____
_____
_____
_____
_____
_____
_____
_____
_____
_____
_____
_____
_____

Radiation Poisoning

Weapon
CDC category: radiation

Alternate Names
Dirty bomb

Etiology
Radiation or fissionable material including
>   Americium-241 (Am-241)
>   Cesium-137 (Ce-137)
>   Cobalt-60 (Co-60)
>   Iodine-131 (I-131)
>   Iridium-192 (Ir-192)
>   Plutonium-238 (Pu-238)
>   Polonium 210 (Po-210)
>   Strontium-90 (Sr-90)

DNA damage causing abnormalities in body chemical and physiological reactions

Transmission
Source:	Industrial, medical
Entry:	Ingestion
	Inhalation
Human-to-Human:	No

Predisposing/Comorbid Conditions
NA

Demographics
Location:	Global
Populations:	All persons with job-related exposure to radio-active materials
Calendar:	Year-round

Systems

Gastrointestinal
Hematopoietic/Immune
Oropharynx
Skin

Incubation

NA

Signs/Symptoms

Abdomen – pain
Appetite – decreased (anorexia)
Arterial press – low (hypotension)
Bowel movements – blood (melena)
Bowel movements – diarrhea
Consciousness – loss, sudden (syncope)
Dehydration
Extremities – pain, shooting (paresthesias)
Eyes, conjunctivae – injected
Fatigue
Hair, local – loss
Hair, gen – loss
Mentation – confusion [1]
Mentation – weak (malaise)
Mouth, gingiva – bleeding
Mouth, gingiva – ulcers
Mouth, mucosa – ulcers
Muscles – weak
Nausea
Nose, mucosa – ulcers
Nose – bleed (epistaxis)
Salivation – increased (psyalism)
Skin, local – burn
Skin, local – inflammation
Skin, local – pain
Skin, local – shedding (desquamation)
Skin, local – vesicles
Skin, sensation local – heat
Skin – bruising
Skin color – red (erythema)

Skin – rash, petechiae
Sweating – increased (hyperhydrosis)
Vomiting
Vomiting – blood (hematemesis)

Differentiation
Includes, but not limited to:
Acute infectious syndrome
Other causes of bone marrow suppression and bleeding

Complications
Include, but not limited to:
Bleeding
Cataracts [1]
Coma
Gastrointestinal toxicity
Hypothyroidism
Microcephaly and mental retardation (in utero) [1]
Neoplasms – leukemia, thyroid cancer [1]
Overwhelming infection/sepsis
Pneumonia
Renal failure

Laboratory
Blood Hgb/Hct – decreased (anemia)
Blood platelets – decreased (thrombocytopenia)
Blood WBC – decreased (leukopenia)

ECG
NA in absence of complications

Imaging
NA in absence of complications

Other Tests
NA in absence of complications

Treatment – Nonpharmacologic
Fluids and electrolytes
Remove clothing
Skin washing ▲

Treatment – Pharmacologic
Antibiotics

Chelation
DTPA
Neupogen
Potassium iodide
Prussian blue

Treatment – Surgical/Invasive

Bone marrow transplant
Burn care

Precautions

Protective clothing: yes
Site decontamination: yes
Other: NS

Primary Prevention

Industrial safety

Course

Varies with exposure intensity

Note

[1]   Very serious exposure

http://www.argus1.com/?radiation

Updates

_____
_____
_____
_____
_____
_____
_____
_____
_____
_____
_____
_____
_____
_____

Ricin Poisoning

Weapon
CDC hazardous chemical category: biotoxin

Alternate Names
NA

Etiology
Protein toxin from castor plant (*ricinus communis*) beans

Inhibits protein synthesis, causing systemic effects and local effects:
　　Airway inflammation, interstitial pneumonia, and perivascular and alveolar edema
　　GI wall inflammation and cell death
　　Muscle and local lymph node cell death

Transmission
Source:	Castor plant
Entry:	Ingestion
	Inhalation
	Injection [1]
Human-to-Human:	No

Predisposing/Comorbid Conditions
NA

Demographics
Location:	Global
Populations:	All
Calendar:	Year-round

Systems
Gastrointestinal
Musculoskeletal
Optic

Respiratory – lower
Respiratory – upper
Skin

Incubation
Hours-days

Signs/Symptoms
Abdomen – pain [2]
Bowel movements – blood or black (melena)
Bowel movements – diarrhea
Breathing – diff, rest (rest dyspnea)
Chest, ant – pain, nonpleuritic rest
Chest – crackles (rales)
Chest – pain/tightness
Cough – acute NS
Eyes, conjunctivae – injected
Eyes, lids – swollen (edema)
Eyes, tearing – increased (lacrimation)
Eyes – pain
Fatigue
Head – pain (headache)
Joints – pain (arthralgia)
Lymph nodes, regional – enlarged
Mentation – hallucination
Muscles, local – pain
Muscles, local – swelling
Muscles, neck – pain
Muscles – pain (myalgia)
Nausea
Seizures
Skin, local – blisters
Skin, local – pain
Skin color – blue (cyanosis)
Skin color – red (erythema)
Skin turgor – decreased
Sweating – increased (hyperhydrosis)
Temperature, body – elevated (fever)
Throat – sore
Urine – blood (hematuria)
Vomiting

Differentiation

Includes, but not limited to:
  Congestive heart failure
  Myocardial infarction
  Phosgene poisoning
  Plague
  Pneumonia
  Pulmonary embolism
  Q fever
  Tularemia

Complications

Include, but not limited to:
  Corneal injury
  Hepatic failure
  Hypovolemia
  Noncardiac pulmonary edema
  Respiratory failure

Laboratory

  Blood arterial pH – decreased (acidosis)
  Blood arterial pO_2 – decreased (hypoxia)
  Blood liver enzymes – increased
  Blood WBC – increased (leukocytosis)
  Urine RBC – present (hematuria, microhematuria)

ECG

  NA in absence of complications

Imaging

  Lungs, parenchyma – infiltrates

Other Tests

  NA in absence of complications

Treatment – Nonpharmacologic

  Eye/skin irrigation and washing ▲

Remove clothing immediately ▲
Ventilation with oxygen

Treatment – Pharmacologic

Antidote: no
NS

Treatment – Surgical/Invasive

NA in absence of complications

Precautions

Protective clothing:	yes
Site decontamination:	yes
Other:	NS

Primary Prevention

Vaccine: in development

Course

Variable
Highly lethal, especially children ☠

Notes

[1] Intentional transmission, i.e., murder
[2] Varies with exposure route

http://www.argus1.com/?ricin

Updates

_____
_____
_____
_____
_____
_____
_____
_____
_____
_____
_____
_____

Riot Control Agents Poisoning

Weapon
CDC hazardous chemical category: riot control agents/tear gas

Alternate Names
NA

Etiology
Agents include:
>>> Bromobenzylcyanide
>>> Chloroacetophenone
>>> Chlorobenzylidenemalononitrile
>>> Chloropicrin
>>> Dibenzoxazepine
>>> Others
Direct irritant to exposed mucosal surfaces

Transmission
Source:	Law enforcement weapons
Entry:	Contact
	Inhalation
Human-to-Human:	No

Predisposing/Comorbid Condition
NA

Demographics
Location:	Global
Populations:	All
Calendar:	Year-round

Systems [1]
Optic
Oropharynx

Respiratory – upper
Skin

Time to Clinical Onset
Immediate

Signs/Symptoms [1]
Breathing – difficult (dyspnea)
Chest – pain/burning
Choking
Cough – acute NS
Eyes, conjunctivae – injected
Eyes, muscles – spasm (blepharospasm)
Eyes, tearing (lacrimation) – increased, excess
Eyes – pain
Mouth, palate – pain/burning
Mouth, salivation – increased (psyalism)
Nose, drainage – increased (rhinorrhea, coryza)
Nose – sneezing
Skin color – red (erythema)
Skin – pain/burning
Throat, swallowing – gagging
Throat – burning
Tongue – pain

Differentiation
Includes, but not limited to:
Other toxic chemical exposures

Complications
Include, but not limited to:
Hypersensitivity reaction

Laboratory
NA in absence of complications

ECG
NA in absence of complications

Imaging
NA in absence of complications

Other Tests
NA in absence of complications

Treatment – Nonpharmacologic
NS

Treatment – Pharmacologic
Antidote: no
NS

Treatment – Surgical/Invasive
NA

Precautions
NA

Primary Prevention
Weapon handling precautions

Course
Short
Variable with exposure intensity and perhaps other factors

Note
[1]   Irritation of exposed mucosal surfaces

http://www.argus1.com/?riot

Updates

_____
_____
_____
_____
_____
_____
_____
_____
_____
_____
_____
_____
_____
_____

Sarin Poisoning

Weapon
CDC hazardous chemical category: nerve agent

Alternate Names
GB

Etiology
Sarin [10]

Cholinesterase inhibition causing widespread neurologic deficits, esp muscle and CNS function

Transmission
Source:	Military weapon arsenal
Entry:	Ingestion
	Inhalation
	Contact
Human-to-Human:	No

Predisposing/Comorbid Conditions
NA

Demographics
Location:	Global
Populations:	All
Calendar:	Year-round

Systems
Nervous
Optic

Time to Clinical Onset
Immediate – hours

Signs/Symptoms

Abdomen – pain

Arterial press – elevated

Arterial press – low (hypotension)

Bowel movements, control – loss [1]

Bowel movements – diarrhea

Breathing – cessation [1]

Breathing – diff, rest (rest dyspnea)

Breathing – rapid (tachypnea)

Chest – pain/tightness

Consciousness – loss, prolonged (coma) [1]

Consciousness – loss, sudden (syncope) [1]

Cough – acute NS

Eyes, conjunctivae – injected [2]

Eyes, pupils – constricted (miosis)

Eyes, tearing (lacrimation) – increased [2]

Eyes, vision – blurred

Eyes, vision – dim

Eyes – pain [2]

Gait – unsteady [1]

Head – pain (headache)

Heart rate – decreased (bradycardia)

Heart rate – increased (tachycardia)

Mentation, judgement – impaired [5]

Mentation, memory – impaired (amnesia) [5]

Mentation – confusion [5]

Mentation – sleepy (somnolence) [5]

Mentation – weak (malaise) [5]

Mood – anxious [5]

Mood – depressed [5]

Mood – restless/irritable [5]

Mouth – drooling

Muscles, movements local – fasciculations

Muscles – paralysis [3]

Muscles – weak

Nausea

Nose, drainage – increased (rhinorrhea, coryza)

Nose – congested

Seizures [1]

Skin, local – sweating [4]

Speech – slurred
Sweating – increased (hyperhydrosis)
Throat – pain/tightness
Urination, spontaneous control – decreased/absent (urinary incontinence)
Urination – frequent (polyuria)
Vomiting

Differentiation
Includes, but not limited to:
Other nerve agent (organophosphate) poisonings

Complications
Include, but not limited to:
Coma
Paralysis
Respiratory failure

Laboratory
Blood arterial pH – increased [8]
Blood cholinesterase – decreased [9]
Blood creatine kinase (CK) – increased [7]
Blood WBC – increased (leukocytosis) [6]

ECG
Dysrhythmias – slow-rate (bradyarrhythmias)
Rate – decreased (sinus bradycardia)
Rate – increased (sinus tachycardia)

Imaging
NS in absence of complications

Other Tests
NS in absence of complications

Treatment – Nonpharmacologic
Do not induce vomiting for ingestion ▲
Remove clothing immediately ▲
Skin/eye washing and irrigation immediately ▲

Treatment – Pharmacologic

Antidotes:

Atropine

Pralidoxime chloride

Treatment – Surgical/Invasive

NA in absence of complications

Precautions

Protective clothing:	yes
Site decontamination:	yes
Other:	SCBA

Primary Prevention

NA

Course

Death usual with severe exposure ☠

Recovery usual with mild or moderate exposure

Survival usual with prompt treatment

Notes

[1]   Severe poisoning

[2]   Local eye symptoms have rapid onset after exposure (seconds to minutes)

[3]   Flaccid

[4]   Area of contact

[5]   CNS manifestations may persist for several weeks after acute effects end

[6]   60% of cases in 1995 Tokyo subway attack

[7]   10% of cases in 1995 Tokyo subway attack

[8]   Respiratory alkalosis; >60% of cases in 1995 Tokyo subway attack

[9]   >50% of cases in 1995 Tokyo subway attack, increases with severity of exposure

[10]   Colorless, odorless, tasteless liquid

http://www.argus1.com/?sarin

Updates

_____

_____

_____

_____

_____

_____

_____

_____

_____

_____

_____

_____

_____

_____

_____

_____

_____

_____

Sodium Monofluoroacetate Poisoning

Weapon
CDC hazardous chemical category: blood agent

Alternate Names
Compound 1080
SMFA

Etiology
Sodium monofluoroacetate ($NaFC_2H_3O_2$)

Internally converted to fluoroacetate, which may block citrate in Krebs cycle inhibiting cell metabolism, but this mechanism has been challenged

Transmission
Source:	Plants, pesticides, military weapon (?)
Entry:	Ingestion
Human-to-Human:	No

Predisposing/Comorbid Condition
NA

Demographics
Location:	Global, esp tropics
Populations:	All, esp farmers
Calendar:	Year-round

Systems
Cardiovascular
Nervous

Time to Clinical Onset
$^1/_2$ hour-20 hours

Signs/Symptoms
Arterial press – low
Breathing – slow
Consciousness – loss, prolonged (coma)
Consciousness – loss, sudden (syncope)
Dizziness (lightheaded)
Heart rhythm – irregular
Nausea
Seizures
Vomiting

Differentiation
Includes, but not limited to:
Acute myocardial infarction
Other causes of CNS depression

Complications
Include, but not limited to:
Dysrhythmias
Respiratory failure
Shock

Laboratory
Blood arterial pH – decreased (acidosis)
Blood calcium – decreased
Blood creatinine – increased
Blood potassium – decreased

ECG
Dysrhythmias, NS
ST-T wave – NS changes

Imaging
NA in absence of complications

Other Tests
NA in absence of complications

Treatment – Nonpharmacologic
Fluids and electrolytes
Gastric lavage
Ventilation

Treatment – Pharmacologic
Antidote: no
Activated charcoal
Cathartics

Treatment – Surgical/Invasive
NA

Precautions
NA

Primary Prevention
NA

Course
Variable, often fatal ☠

http://www.argus1.com/?sodiummono

Updates

_____
_____
_____
_____
_____
_____
_____
_____
_____
_____
_____

Sulfuryl Fluoride Poisoning

Weapon
CDC hazardous chemical category: choking/lung/pulmonary agent

Alternate Names
Profume
Sulfonyl fluoride
Sulfur dioxide difluoride
Sulfuryl difluoride
Sulphuryl fluoride
Vikane
Zythor

Etiology
Sulfuryl fluoride (SO_2F_2) [2]

Generates fluoride ion when metobolized in tissue or hydrolyzed in water

Transmission
Source:	Industrial insecticides and rodenticides
Entry:	Inhalation
Human-to-Human:	No

Predisposing/Comorbid Condition
NA

Demographics
Location:	Global, esp agricultural areas
Populations:	All, esp pesticide handlers
Calendar:	Year-round

Systems
Nervous
Oropharynx
Respiratory – upper

Time to Clinical Onset
Immediate

Signs/Symptoms
Abdomen – pain
Breathing – diff, acute (acute dyspnea)
Breathing – rapid (tachypnea)
Breath sounds – crackling (rales)
Breath sounds – wheezes
Cough – acute NS
Eyes, conjunctivae – injected
Eyes – irritation
Eyes – tearing, excess (lacrimation)
Gait – abnormal (ataxia)
Mentation – depression
Mentation – weakness (malaise)
Mood – restless, irritable
Mouth – burning
Muscle movement – slow voluntary
Muscles – twitching
Nausea
Nose – irritation
Seizures
Speech – slow
Throat – burning
Vomiting

Differentiation
Includes, but not limited to:
Other causes of acute respiratory distress
Other causes of CNS depression

Complications
Include, but not limited to:
Liver necrosis
Noncardiac pulmonary edema
Pulmonary necrosis
Renal necrosis

Laboratory
Blood calcium – decreased
Blood fluoride – elevated [1]
Blood potassium – decreased

ECG
NA in absence of complications

Imaging
NA in absence of complications

Other Tests
NA in absence of complications

Treatment – Nonpharmacologic
Fluids and electrolytes
Ventilation

Treatment – Pharmacologic
Antidote: no
NS

Treatment – Surgical/Invasive
NA

Precautions
NA

Primary Prevention
Home fumigation precautions
Industrial precautions

Course
Variable

Notes
[1]   Not diagnostic – varies with diet, environment exposures
[2]   Colorless, odorless gas

http://www.argus1.com/?sufuryl

Updates

Sulfur Mustard Poisoning

Weapon
CDC hazardous chemical category: blister agent/vessicant

Alternate Names
"H"
"HD"
"HT"
Mustard gas
Mustard agent

Etiology
Sulfur mustard [2]

Alkylating agent with cholinergic and other undefined mechanisms

Transmission
Source:	Military weapon
Entry:	Contact
	Inhalation
Human-to-Human:	No

Predisposing/Comorbid Condition
NA

Demographics
Location:	Global
Populations:	All
Calendar:	NA

Systems
Optic
Respiratory – upper
Respiratory – lower
Skin

Time to Clinical Onset
4-24 hours

Signs/Symptoms
Abdomen – pain
Bowel movements – diarrhea
Breathing – diff, acute (acute dyspnea)
Breath sounds – coarse (rhonchi, general)
Breath sounds – crackling (rales)
Breath sounds – wheezes
Chest – pain, burning
Cough – acute NS
Cough – productive
Eyes, conjunctivae – injected
Eyes, cornea – ulcer
Eyes, lids – edema
Eyes, pupils – constricted (miosis)
Eyes, vision – light sensitivity, increased (photophobia)
Eyes, vision – loss
Eyes – irritation
Eyes – pain
Eyes – tearing, excess (lacrimation)
Nausea
Nose – blood (epistaxis)
Nose – discharge (rhinorrhea)
Nose – sneezing
Prostration
Skin – blisters [1]
Skin color – erythema [1]
Skin – itching (pruritus) [1]
Temperature, body – elevated (fever)
Voice – hoarse
Voice – loss
Vomiting

Differentiation
Includes, but not limited to:
Other blistering agents

Complications
Include, but not limited to:
Blindness
Cornea ulcer/perforation
Noncardiac pulmonary edema
Pneumonia
Skin 2nd and 3rd degree burns

Laboratory
NS in absence of complications

Imaging
NS in absence of complications

Other Tests
NS in absence of complications

Treatment – Nonpharmacologic
Do not induce vomiting ▲
Do not cover eyes with bandages ▲
Fluids and electrolytes
Immediate clothing removal ▲
Immediate eye and skin irrigation/washing ▲
Ventilation

Treatment – Pharmacologic
Antidote: no
NS

Treatment – Surgical/Invasive
NA

Precautions
Protective clothing: yes
Site decontamination: yes
Other: SCBA

Primary Prevention
NA

Course

Mortality with treatment <5%

Notes

[1]   Warm, moist, thin skin most vulnerable
[2]   Yellow-brown liquid with garlic or mustard odor

http://www.argus1.com/?mustard

Updates

_____
_____
_____
_____
_____
_____
_____
_____
_____
_____
_____
_____
_____
_____
_____
_____
_____
_____
_____

Super Warfarin Poisoning

Weapon
CDC hazardous chemical category: long-acting anticoagulant

Alternate Names
Brodifacoum (most common form)

Etiology
Hydroxycoumarin

Decreases activity of vitamin K-dependent blood clotting factors II, VII, IX, and X

Transmission
Source:	Rodent poisons
Entry:	Ingestion
Human-to-Human:	No

Predisposing/comorbid conditions
Major depression [2]
Existing anticoagulation

Demographics
Location:	Global
Populations:	All, esp children and persons with Munchausen syndrome [4]
Calendar:	Year-round

System
Coagulation

Time to Clinical Onset
24-72 hours [3]

Signs/Symptoms

Bowel movements – blood or black (hematochezia) (melena)
Mouth, gingiva – bleeding
Nose – blood (epistaxis)
Skin – ecchymoses
Skin – rash, petechiae
Sputum – blood (hemoptysis)
Urine – blood (hematuria)
Vagina – blood
Vomiting – blood (hematemesis)

Differentiation

Includes, but not limited to:
All coagulopathies
Viral hemorrhagic fevers

Complications

Include, but not limited to:
Acute blood loss
Intracranial hemorrhage

Laboratory

Blood factor II – decreased
Blood factor VII – decreased
Blood factor IX – decreased
Blood factor X – decreased
Blood partial thromboplastin time (PTT) – increased
Blood prothrombin time (PT) – increased
Blood-specific detection – present

ECG

NA in absence of complications

Imaging

NA in absence of complications

Other Tests

Drug-specific detection in environmental samples

Treatment – Nonpharmacologic
Blood, whole or fresh plasma [1]
Gastric lavage
Induce vomiting

Treatment – Pharmacologic
Antidote: phytonadione (vitamin K1)
Charcoal absorption

Treatment – Surgical/Invasive
NA in absence of complications

Precautions
NA

Primary Prevention
Place rodenticides out of reach of children ▲

Course
Variable with intensity of exposure and timeliness of treatment

Notes
[1]   For hemorrhage
[2]   Suicide attempts
[3]   Effects last days-months
[4]   May be difficult to diagnose in these persons

http://www.argus1.com/?superwarf

Updates

_____
_____
_____
_____
_____
_____
_____
_____
_____
_____
_____
_____
_____

Tabun Poisoning

Weapon
CDC hazardous chemical category: nerve agent

Alternate Names
GA

Etiology
Tabun [7]

Acts by cholinergic stimulation

Transmission
Source:	Military arsenal
Entry:	Contact
	Inhalation
Human-to-Human:	No

Predisposing/Comorbid Conditions
NA

Demographics
Location:	Global
Populations:	All
Calendar:	Year-round

Systems
Nervous
Optic

Time to Clinical Onset
Vapor: seconds
Liquid: hours

Signs/Symptoms

Abdomen – pain
Arterial press – decreased (hypotension)
Arterial press – increased
Bowel movements, control – decrease/loss [1]
Bowel movements – diarrhea
Breathing – cessation [1]
Breathing – diff, rest (rest dyspnea)
Breathing – rapid (tachypnea)
Chest – pain/tightness
Consciousness – loss, prolonged (coma) [1]
Consciousness – loss, sudden (syncope) [1]
Cough – acute NS
Eyes, conjunctivae – injected [2]
Eyes, pupils – constricted (miosis) [6]
Eyes, tearing – increased (lacrimation) [2]
Eyes, vision – blurred
Eyes, vision – dim
Eyes – pain [2]
Gait – unsteady [1]
Head – pain (headache)
Heart rate – decreased (bradycardia)
Heart rate – increased (tachycardia)
Mentation, judgement – impaired [5]
Mentation, memory – impaired (amnesia) [5]
Mentation – confusion [5]
Mentation – sleepy (somnolence) [5]
Mentation – weak (malaise) [5]
Mood – anxious [5]
Mood – depressed [5]
Mood – restless/irritable [5]
Mouth – drooling
Muscles, local – movement, fine (fasciculations)
Muscles – paralysis [3]
Muscles – weak
Nausea
Nose, drainage – increased (rhinorrhea, coryza)
Nose – congestion
Seizures [1]
Skin, local – sweating [4]

Skin, local – twitching (fasciculations) [4]
Speech – slurred
Sweating – increased (hyperhydrosis)
Throat – pain/tightness
Urination, control – decreased/absent (urinary incontinence) [1]
Urination – frequent (polyuria)
Vomiting

Differentiation
Includes, but not limited to:
Sarin poisoning
Soman poisoning
VX poisoning

Complications
Include, but not limited to:
Coma
Paralysis
Respiratory failure

Laboratory
Blood arterial pH – increased
Blood cholinesterase – decreased
Blood creatine kinase (CK) – increased
Blood WBC – increased (leukocytosis)

ECG
Rate – rapid (sinus tachycardia)
Rate – slow (sinus bradycardia)

Imaging
NA in absence of complications

Other Tests
NA in absence of complications

Treatment – Nonpharmacologic
Airway maintenance
Eye/skin irrigation and washing immediately ▲
Immediate triage if cardiac activity present in absence of breathing ▲
Remove victim from source as soon as possible

Treatment – Pharmacologic

Antidote: atropine

Anticonvulsant

Treatment – Surgical/Invasive

NA in absence of complications

Precautions

Protective clothing:	yes
Site decontamination:	yes
Other:	NS

Primary Prevention

NA

Course

Variable with intensity of exposure

Notes

[1] Severe poisoning

[2] Local eye symptoms have rapid onset after exposure (seconds to minutes)

[3] Flaccid

[4] Area of contact

[5] CNS manifestations may persist for several weeks after acute effects end

[6] Usually bilateral; may be unilateral

[7] Clear, colorless, tasteless

http://www.argus1.com/?tabun

Updates

_____

_____

_____

_____

_____

_____

_____

_____

_____

_____

_____

Tetrodotoxin Poisoning

Weapon
CDC hazardous chemical category: biotoxin

Alternate Names
Fugu poisoning [4]
Pufferfish poisoning

Etiology
Tetrodotoxin ($C_{11}H_{17}N_3O_8$) [3]

Selective blockade of fast sodium channels in nerves and muscle
membranes

Transmission
Source:	Pufferfish
Entry:	Ingestion
Human-to-Human:	No

Predisposing/Comorbid Conditions
NA

Demographics
Location:	Global, coasts
Populations:	All
Calendar:	Year-round, sporadic

Systems
Gastrointestinal
Nervous

Time to Clinical Onset
Minutes

Signs/Symptoms
Abdomen – pain

Arterial press – low [2]
Bowel movements – diarrhea
Cranial nerves – palsy
Dizziness (true vertigo)
Extremities – pain, shooting (paresthesias)
Extremities – sensations, abnormal (dysesthesias)
Head – pain (headache)
Heart rate – slow (bradycardia)
Mentation – floating sensation
Mouth – numb
Muscles, gen – paralysis
Muscles – pain (myalgia)
Muscles – weak
Nausea
Seizures
Sensations, abnormal (dysesthesias) [1]
Skin – sensation, reversed hot-cold
Speech – inarticulate (dysarthria)
Sweating – increased (hyperhydrosis)
Vomiting

Differentiation
Includes, but not limited to:
Saxitoxin and other neurotoxins

Complications
Include, but not limited to:
Cardiac dysrhythmias
Respiratory failure
Shock

Laboratory
NA in absence of complications

ECG
NA in absence of complications

Imaging
NA in absence of complications

Other Tests
NA in absence of complications

Treatment – Nonpharmacologic
Cardiac pacemaker [5]
Fluids and electrolytes
Ventilation

Treatment – Pharmacologic
Antidote: no
NS

Treatment – Surgical/Invasive
NA

Precautions
NA

Primary Prevention
Cooking does not inactivate tetrodotoxin ▲
Public health control of exposure to toxic shellfish

Course
>50% mortality in Japan ☠

Notes
[1]   Esp lips, mouth, upper airways, fingers within minutes of ingestion
[2]   Due to weak hypotensive effect
[3]   Synthesized by bacteria *pseudomonas tetraodonis* and other species in shellfish
[4]   Japan, where tetrodotoxin is the major cause of death due to food poisoning ☠
[5]   Bradyarrhythmias

http://www.argus1.com/?tetrodotoxin

Updates

_____

_____

_____

_____

_____

_____

_____

_____

_____

_____

_____

_____

_____

_____

_____

_____

_____

_____

_____

_____

Thallium Poisoning

Weapon
CDC hazardous chemical category: metal

Alternate Names
NA

Etiology
Thallium [3]

Disrupts sodium-potassium ATP, esp in mitochrondia

Transmission [6]
Source:	Rodenticides; electronic and chemical research
Entry:	Ingestion
	Inhalation
Human-to-Human:	No

Predisposing/Comorbid Conditions
NA

Demographics
Location:	Global
Populations:	All
Calendar:	Year-round

Systems
Cardiovascular
Gastrointestinal
Nervous
Optic
Skin

Time to Clinical Onset
Hours

Signs/Symptoms [1]

Abdomen – pain [1]
Arterial press – elevated [8]
Bowel movements – constipation [5]
Bowel movements – diarrhea [4]
Bowel movements – blood or black (hematochezia) (melena)
Chest, ant – pain/pressure/burning [8]
Consciousness – loss, prolonged (coma)
Extremities, feet – footdrop [10]
Extremities, hands/nails – Aldrich-Mees lines [11]
Extremities, hands/palms – red (palmar erythema)
Extremities – abnormal sensations (dysesthesias) [1, 2]
Extremities – tremors [10]
Extremities – weakness
Eyes, lids – drooping (ptosis) [1]
Eyes, retina/optic nerve – inflammation
Eyes, vision/binocular – loss, total (blindness)
Eyes, vision – loss, spotty (scotoma)
Eyes, vision – loss, subtotal
Gait – ataxic [1]
Hair – loss [1]
Hair – pigmentation, increased
Heart rate – increased (tachycardia) [8]
Lips – ulcers
Mentation – confusion
Mentation – memory impaired (amnesia) [10]
Mentation – psychosis
Mouth, gingiva pigmentation – increased
Nausea
Seizures
Skin – rash, nonspecific
Vomiting

Differentiation

Includes, but not limited to:
Acute porphyria
Antimony poisoning
Arsenic poisoning
Guillain-Barré syndrome

Other polyneuropathies
Selenosis

Complications
Include, but not limited to:
Respiratory failure [9]

Laboratory
Blood Hgb/Hct – decreased (anemia)
Blood liver enzymes – increased
Blood platelets – decreased (thrombocytopenia)
Blood thallium – positive
Stool blood – present
Urine thallium – positive

ECG
Rate – rapid (sinus tachycardia) [8]
T wave – inversion, abnormal [8]

Imaging
NA in absence of complications

Other Tests
Electroretinography
Electromyogram
Nerve biopsy – demyelination

Treatment – Nonpharmacologic
NS

Treatment – Pharmacologic
Binding agents
activated charcoal
ferric ferrocyanide
Diuresis
Enhanced fecal excretion
Hemodialysis
Hemoperfusion
Prussian blue [7]

Treatment – Surgical/Invasive
NA in absence of complications

Precautions
NA

Primary Prevention
NA

Course
Variable

Death may occur 1-2 weeks after exposure ☠

Notes
[1] Clinical triad of gastroenteritis, hair loss, peripheral neuropathy

[2] Esp hyperesthesia of soles

[3] Heavy metal similar to potassium

[4] Early in course

[5] Late in course

[6] Also a homicidal agent

[7] Reduces enterohepatic circulation

[8] Cardiovascular signs begin about 1 week after clinical onset

[9] Due to neuropathy

[10] Residual stage about 4 weeks after onset

[11] White bands

http://www.argus1.com/?thallium

Updates

_____

_____

_____

_____

_____

_____

_____

_____

_____

_____

_____

Trichothecene Poisoning

Classification
CDC hazardous chemical category: biotoxin

Alternate Names
Mycotoxins
T2
Yellow rain

Etiology
Trichothecene mycotoxin [1]

Inhibits synthesis of protein and nucleic acid

Transmission
Source:	Grains, mushrooms
Entry:	Contact
	Ingestion
	Inhalation
Human-to-Human:	No

Predisposing/Comorbid Condition
NA

Demographics
Location:	Global [2]
Populations:	All
Calendar:	Year-round

Systems
Coagulation
Gastrointestinal
Respiratory – upper
Skin

Time to Clinical Onset
Minutes

Signs/Symptoms

Abdomen – pain
Appetite – reduced (anorexia)
Arterial press – low [3]
Bowel movements, stool – blood or black (hematochezia) (melena)
Bowel movements – diarrhea
Breathing – diff, acute (acute dyspnea)
Breathing – rapid (tachypnea)
Breath sounds, gen – wheezes
Cough – acute NS
Dizziness (lightheaded)
Eyes, conjunctivae – injected
Eyes, vision – blurred
Eyes – pain
Eyes – tearing, excess (lacrimation)
Gait – ataxic
Heart rate – rapid (tachycardia) [3]
Mentation – weakness (malaise)
Mouth – pain/burning
Nausea
Nose – bleeding (epistaxis)
Nose – drainage (rhinorrhea, coryza)
Nose – irritation
Nose – pain
Nose – sneezing
Saliva – blood
Skin, gen – blisters
Skin, gen – necrosis, sloughing
Skin, gen – pain, burning
Skin, gen – rash, erythematous
Skin, gen – tender
Temperature, body – decreased (hypothermia) [3]
Vomiting

Differentiation

Includes, but not limited to:
Other causes of acute multisystem disease

Complications
Include, but not limited to:
   Coagulopathy
   Multi-organ failure

Laboratory
   Environmental detection of agent
   Otherwise NS

Imaging
   NA in absence of complications

Other Tests
   NA in absence of complications

Treatment – Nonpharmacologic
   NS

Treatment – Pharmacologic
   Antidote: no
   NS

Treatment – Surgical/Invasive
   NA

Precautions
   Protective clothing: yes
   Site decontamination: yes
   Other: SCBA

Primary Prevention
   Vaccine: no

Course
   Variable with exposure route and intensity
   Death may occur in minutes-days ☠

Notes
[1]   Produced by molds of genera *trichoderma*, *fusarium*, *myrotecium*, and others
[2]   Suspected bioweapon use in 1970s and 80s in SE Asia and Afghanistan
[3]   Preterminal

http://www.argus1.com/?trichothecene

Updates

_____

_____

_____

_____

_____

_____

_____

_____

_____

_____

_____

_____

_____

_____

_____

_____

_____

_____

_____

VX Poisoning

Classification
CDC hazardous chemical category: nerve agent

Alternate Names
NA

Etiology
Methylphosphonothiolate ($C_{11}H_{26}NO_2PS$)

Cholinergic stimulation

Transmission
Source:	Military weapon
Entry:	Contact
	Inhalation
Human-to-Human:	No

Predisposing/Comorbid Conditions
NA

Demographics
Location:	Global
Population:	All
Time:	Year-round

Systems
Nervous

Time to Clinical Onset
Seconds (vapor form) to hours depending on dose

Signs/Symptoms
Abdomen – cramps
Arterial press – elevated
Arterial press – low (hypotension)

Bowel movements, control – decreased/absent [1]
Bowel movements – diarrhea
Breathing, rate – increased (tachypnea)
Breathing – cessation [1]
Breathing – difficult, acute (dyspnea)
Chest – pain/burning/tightness
Consciousness – loss, prolonged (coma) [1]
Consciousness – loss, sudden (syncope) [1]
Cough – acute NS
Eyes, pupils – constricted (miosis)
Eyes, tearing (lacrimation) – increased
Eyes, vision – blurred
Eyes, vision – dim
Eyes – pain
Gait – unsteady [1]
Head – pain (headache)
Heart rate – decreased (bradycardia)
Heart rate – increased (tachycardia)
Mentation – confusion
Mentation – sleepy (somnolence)
Mouth – drooling
Muscles – twitching
Muscles – weak
Nausea
Nose, drainage – increased (rhinorrhea, coryza)
Nose – congested
Seizures [1]
Skin, sweating – increased (hyperhydrosis)
Urination, control – decreased/lost (incontinence) [1]
Urination, frequency – increased (polyuria)
Vomiting

Differentiation
Includes, but not limited to:
Other nerve agents

Complications
Include, but not limited to:
Coma
Death ☠

Laboratory

NS in absence of complications

ECG

Rate – rapid (sinus tachycardia)
Rate – slow (sinus bradycardia)

Imaging

NS in absence of complications

Other Tests

NA in absence of complications

Treatment – Nonpharmacologic

Do not induce vomiting ▲
Eye/skin irrigation and washing immediately▲
Remove clothing immediately ▲
Ventilation

Treatment – Pharmacologic

Antidote: atropine

Treatment – Surgical/Invasive

NA

Precautions

Protective clothing:	yes
Site decontamination:	yes
Other:	SCBA

Primary Prevention

NA

Course

Variable, including death depending on exposure ☠

Note

[1]   Severe exposure

http://www.argus1.com/?vx

Updates

_____
_____
_____
_____
_____
_____
_____
_____
_____
_____
_____
_____
_____
_____
_____
_____
_____
_____
_____
_____
_____
_____

CLINICAL GUIDE— ACUTE COMPLICATIONS

Adrenal Failure

Note: In addition to the conditions listed, all other agents that cause septic shock can also cause secondary acute adrenal failure by direct tissue damage to the adrenal or pituitary gland.

Alternate Names
Acute adrenal crisis

Clinical Guide Primary Conditions
Any cause of acute adrenal hemorrhage
Leptospirosis [5]
Meningococcemia [5]

Signs/Symptoms
Abdomen, flank – pain
Abdomen – pain
Appetite – decreased (anorexia)
Arterial press – low
Breathing – rapid (tachypnea)
Chills
Consciousness – loss, prolonged (coma)
Consciousness – loss, sudden (syncope)
Dizziness (lightheaded)
Fatigue
Head – pain (headache)
Heart rate – rapid (tachycardia)
Mentation – confused
Muscles – movement, slow/sluggish
Muscles – weak [1]
Nausea
Skin – rash, nonspecific
Skin turgor – decreased (dehydration)

Sweating – increased (hyperhydrosis) [3]
Temperature, body – elevated (fever) [2]
Weight – loss
Vomiting

Laboratory

Blood cortisol – decreased
Blood glucose – decreased (hypoglycemia)
Blood potassium – increased
Blood sodium – decreased

ECG

Rate – rapid (sinus tachycardia)
T wave – peaked [4]

Other Tests

Cortisol administration – clinical improvement

Notes

[1]   May be profound
[2]   May be high
[3]   Esp face, hands
[4]   Due to hyperkalemia
[5]   Acute hemorrhage into adrenal gland

http://www.argus1.com/?adrenal

Updates

_____
_____
_____
_____
_____
_____
_____
_____
_____
_____
_____

Arthritis

Signs/Symptoms

Joint(s) – pain (arthralgia)
Joint(s) – stiffness
Joint(s) – swelling
Joint(s) – tenderness, local
Joint(s) – warmth
Temperature, body – elevated (fever)

http://www.argus1.com/?arthritis

Updates

Congestive Heart Failure

Alternate Names
Acute cardiac decompensation

Clinical Guide Primary Conditions
Arsine poisoning
Ethylene glycol poisoning
Leptospirosis
Meningococcemia
Trichinellosis
Yellow fever

Signs/Symptoms
Abdomen, RUQ – pain
Abdomen – distention
Abdomen – fullness
Abdomen – fluid (ascites)
Appearance, general – wasting (cachexia)
Appetite – decreased (anorexia)
Arterial pressure – low
Arterial pulse – amplitude, alternating (pulsus alternans)
Behavior – changed [1]
Bowel movements – diarrhea
Breathing – diff, acute (acute dyspnea)
Breathing – diff, effort (effort dyspnea)
Breathing – diff, nocturnal (nocturnal dyspnea)
Breathing – diff, reclining flat (orthopnea)
Breathing – diff, rest (rest dyspnea)
Breathing – rapid (tachypnea)
Breathing – rhythmic changes (Cheyne-Stokes)
Breath sounds – crackling (rales)
Breath sounds– decreased

Breath sounds – wheezes
Consciousness – loss, sudden (syncope)
Cough – chronic NS
Cough – nocturnal
Extremities, lower bilat – edema
Eyes – prominent (exophthalmos, proptosis) [2]
Fatigue
Head – pain (headache)
Heart, LV apex – impulse, inferior displacement
Heart, LV apex – impulse, lateral displacement
Heart rate – rapid (tachycardia)
Heart rhythm – irregular [3]
Heart sound P2 – loud
Heart sound – S3 LV
Heart sound – S3 RV
Heart sound – S4 LV
Heart sound – S4 RV
Heart sounds – intensity decreased
Liver – enlarged (hepatomegaly)
Liver – tender
Mentation – confused [1]
Muscles – weak
Nausea
Skin color – blue (cyanosis)
Skin color – yellow (jaundice)
Skin – itching (pruritus)
Sleep – disturbed (insomnia)
Spleen – enlarged (splenomegaly)
Sputum – blood (hemoptysis)
Urination – nighttime (nocturia)
Venous pulse, jugular – abdominojugular reflux
Venous pulse, jugular – elevated
Vomiting
Weight – gain [4]

Laboratory

Blood arterial pO_2 – decreased (hypoxia)
Blood arterial pCO_2 – decreased
Blood BNP – increased ▲ [7]
Blood creatinine – increased

Blood sodium – decreased
Blood urea nitrogen – increased

ECG

Abnormalities – nonspecific and variable
Dysrhythmias, atrial [6]
Dysrhythmias, ventricular
Rate – rapid (sinus tachycardia)

Imaging

Heart – enlarged
Lungs, vasculature – congested

Other Tests

Cardiac catheterization [5]
Echocardiography

Notes

[1]   Esp elderly
[2]   Due to chronic elevation of venous pressure
[3]   Esp atrial fibrillation
[4]   Unexplained
[5]   If primary or contributory cardiac etiology is possible and cannot first
      be resolved by noninvasive tests
[6]   Esp atrial fibrillation
[7]   Differentiation from other, noncardiac causes of acute dyspnea ▲

http://www.argus1.com/?chf

Updates

_____
_____
_____
_____
_____
_____
_____
_____
_____
_____
_____

Corneal Injury

Alternate Names
Cornea ulcer

Clinical Guide Primary Conditions
Ammonia poisoning
Benzene poisoning
Chlorine poisoning
Lewisite
Methyl bromide poisoning
Osmium tetroxide poisoning
Phosgene poisoning
Ricin poisoning
Smallpox
Sulfur mustard poisoning

Signs/Symptoms
Eyes, conjunctivae – injected
Eyes, cornea – ulcer
Eyes, vision – altered, nonspecific
Eyes, vision – light sensitivity, increased (photophobia)
Eyes – tearing, excess (lacrimation)
Eyes – burning, itching (asthenopia)
Eyes – pain

Tests
Cornea flouorescein stain
Keratometry
Pupillary reflex
Refraction
Slit-lamp exam
Tear test
Visual acuity

http://www.argus1.com/?corneainjury

Updates

_____

_____

_____

_____

_____

_____

_____

_____

_____

_____

_____

_____

_____

_____

_____

_____

_____

_____

_____

_____

Dehydration

Note: all causes of fever and/or severe fluid loss can cause dehydration in addition to the agents listed below.

Clinical Guide Primary Conditions

Arsine poisoning
Brevetoxin poisoning
BZ poisoning
Campylobacteriosis
Chickenpox
Cholera
Clostridium perfringens gastroenteritis
Colchicine poisoning
Cryptosporidiosis
E coli 0157:H7
Gastroenteritis – viral
Giardiasis
Ricin poisoning
Salmonellosis
Shigellosis
Smallpox
Staphylococcus food poisoning
Viral gastroenteritis
Yersiniosis

Signs/Symptoms

Arterial press – low
Arterial press – upright, low (orthostatic hypotension)
Consciousness – loss, prolonged (coma)
Eyes, tears – decreased
Eyes – sunken
Head, fontanelles – sunken [1]

Heart rate – rapid (tachycardia)
Mentation – weakness (malaise)
Mood – lethargic
Mouth – dry (xerostomia)
Seizures
Skin capillary refill – delayed
Skin turgor – decreased
Urine – reduced (oliguria)

Laboratory

Blood urea nitrogen – increased [2]
Blood creatinine – increased [2]
Blood Hgb/Hct – increased [2]
Blood sodium – increased [2]
Urine specific gravity – increased
Urine volume – decreased (oliguria)

ECG

Rate – rapid (sinus tachycardia)

Notes

[1]   Infants
[2]   Due to hemoconcentration

http://www.argus1.com/?dehyd

Updates

Disseminated Intravascular Coagulation

Alternate Names
DIC
Purpura fulminans [2]

Clinical Guide **Primary Conditions**
Carbon monoxide poisoning
Chickenpox
Colchicine poisoning
Crimean Congo hemorrhagic fever
Ebola hemorrhagic fever
Legionellosis
Leptospirosis
Listeriosis
Marburg hemorrhagic fever
Meningococcemia
Plague
Psittacosis
Tularemia
Yellow fever

Signs/Symptoms
Bleeding – easy
Extremities, fingers – bluish color [1]

Laboratory
Blood antithrombin – variable

Blood fibrinogen degradation products – increased
Blood fibrinogen – variable
Blood platelets – decreased
Blood prothrombin time – increased

Notes

[1]   Due to thrombosis
[2]   Associated with tissue necrosis

http://www.argus1.com/?dic

Updates

_____
_____
_____
_____
_____
_____
_____
_____
_____
_____
_____
_____
_____
_____
_____
_____
_____
_____
_____
_____

Guillain – Barré Syndrome

Note: the exact mechanism of Guillain-Barré is unknown and can follow many viral and bacterial infections in addition to those listed below.

Alternate Names
Acute infectious polyneuritis
Landry's ascending paralysis
Strohl syndrome

Clinical Guide Primary Conditions
Avian influenza
Campylobacteriosis
Chickenpox
Infectious mononucleosis
Leptospirosis

Signs/Symptoms
Arterial pressure – elevated [1, 7]
Arterial pressure – low [1, 7]
Arterial pressure – upright, low (orthostatic hyp) [7]
Back – pain
Cranial nerves – palsy
Extremities – pain, shooting (paresthesias)
Eyes, motion – reduced or paralyzed (ophthalmoplegia) [2]
Eyes, vision – double (diplopia)
Face, cheeks – flushed
Face, muscles bilat – weak/paralyzed
Heart rate – rapid (tachycardia) [3, 7]
Heart rate – slow (bradycardia) [3, 7]
Muscles, cranial nerve innervated – weakness [4]
Muscles, movement – incoordinated (ataxia) [2]

Muscles, up/low unilat – paralysis (hemiplegia)
Muscles, up/low unilat – weakness (hemiparesis)
Muscles – pain (myalgia) [5]
Muscles – weakness [6]
Sensation, general deep – reduced
Skin – sensation reduced (dysesthesia)
Swallowing – difficult (dysphagia)
Sweating – decreased [7]
Sweating – increased (hyperhydrosis) [7]
Tendon reflexes – reduced or absent
Urination – retention [7]

Laboratory
CSF protein – increased [8]

ECG
Dysrhythmias, atrial
Dysrhythmias, ventricular
Rate – decreased (bradycardia) [3]
Rate – increased (tachycardia) [3]

Other Tests
EMG [9]
Pulmonary function [10]

Notes
[1]   Fluctuating
[2]   Miller-Fisher variant
[3]   Tachycardia more common
[4]   Landry's ascending paralysis
[5]   Esp hips, thighs, back
[6]   Symmetrical proximal and distal muscles; usually lower extremities first; evolves over days
[7]   Disturbance of autonomic function, usually lasts only days
[8]   With normal WBC
[9]   Findings consistent with demyelination
[10]   Determine respiratory neuromuscular capacity

http://www.argus1.com/?gbs

Updates

Hemolytic Anemia

Clinical Guide Primary Conditions
Anthrax
E coli 0157 : H7
Infectious mononucleosis
Phosgene poisoning
Psittacosis

Signs/Symptoms
Breathing – diff, effort (effort dyspnea)
Chills
Fatigue
Heart rate – rapid (tachycardia)
Skin color – pale (palor)
Skin color – yellow (jaundice)
Spleen – enlarged (splenomegaly)
Urine – dark

Laboratory [2]
Blood bilirubin – increased [1]
Blood haptoglobin – decreased
Blood Hgb/Hct – decreased (anemia)
Blood LDH – increased
Blood RBC – decreased
Blood reticulocyte count – increased
Feces urobilinogen – present/increased
Urine hemoglobin – present (hemoglobinuria)
Urine hemosiderin – present
Urine urobilinogen – present/increased

ECG [2]
Rate – rapid (sinus tachycardia)

Note

[1]   Indirect bilirubin

http://www.argus1.com/?hemolytic

Updates

_____
_____
_____
_____
_____
_____
_____
_____
_____
_____
_____
_____
_____
_____
_____
_____
_____
_____
_____
_____

Hepatic Failure

Clinical Guide **Primary Conditions**

Arsenic poisoning
Crimeran-Congo hemorrhagic fever
Ebola hemorrhagic fever
Infectious hepatitis
Leptospirosis
Lewisite poisoning
Malaria
Marburg hemorrhagic fever
Meningococcemia
Methyl bromide poisoning
Phosgene poisoning
Phosphine poisoning
Ricin poisoning
Rift Valley fever
Yellow fever

Signs/Symptoms

Consciousness – loss, prolonged (coma)
Eyes, conjunctivae color – yellow (icterus)
Mentation – confused
Mentation – delirium
Mentation – dementia, fluctuating
Mentation – sleepiness (somnolence)
Mood – labile
Mood – lethargic
Mood – restless/irritable
Muscles, fine motor movement – loss [1]
Muscles – movement, spontaneous
Muscles – stiffness
Muscles – tremor, flappy
Skin color – yellow (icterus)

Speech – disturbed (dysphasia)
Seizures [2]

Laboratory
Blood albumin – decreased
Blood ammonia – increased
Blood bilirubin – increased
Blood prothrombin time – increased [3]

Other Tests
EEG – NS abnormalities

Notes
[1]   Handwriting
[2]   Rare
[3]   Not corrected with Vitamin K

http://www.argus1.com/?hepaticfailure

Updates

_____
_____
_____
_____
_____
_____
_____
_____
_____
_____
_____
_____
_____
_____
_____
_____
_____
_____
_____
_____

Hyperkalemia

Note: in addition to the conditions listed, any cause of adrenal or renal failure, rhabdomyolysis, or hemolytic anemia may cause hyperkalemia.

Clinical Guide Primary Conditions

Anthrax
Arsine poisoning
Ethylene glycol poisoning
Yellow fever

Signs/Symptoms

Arterial pulse, amp – absent or reduced [1] ▲
Heart, rhythm – irregular [1] ▲
Heart rate – slow (bradycardia) [1] ▲
Nausea

Laboratory

Blood potassium – increased

ECG

AV conduction – 3rd degree block
Dysrhythmias, ventricular
Rate – slow (sinus bradycardia)
T wave – peaked

Note

[1] May indicate serious cardiac arrhythmia requiring immediate ECG
     monitoring and treatment ▲

http://www.argus1.com/?hyperkalemia

Updates

Meningitis/Encephalitis

Clinical Guide Primary Conditions

Anthrax
Arsine poisoning
Avian influenza
Brucellosis
Campylobacteriosis
Chickenpox
Cholera
Dengue
Glanders
Infectious hepatitis
Infectious mononucleosis
Influenza
Lassa fever
Leptospirosis
Listeriosis
Lyme disease
Malaria
Meningococcemia
Mercury poisoning
Monkeypox
Mumps
Parvovirus 19
Pertussis
Plague
Psittacosis
Q fever
Rift Valley fever
Rocky Mountain spotted fever
Rubella
Rubeola

Salmonellosis
Smallpox
Streptococcal pharyngitis
Trichinellosis
Tularemia
West Nile fever
Yellow fever
Yersiniosis

Signs/Symptoms

Abdomen – pain
Arterial press, gen – elevated
Bowel movements, control – loss
Bowel movements – diarrhea
Chills
Consciousness – loss, prolonged (coma)
Cranial nerves, general – palsy
Eyes, motion – jerky (nystagmus)
Eyes, motion – reduced or paralyzed (ophthalmoplegia)
Eyes, vision – field defects
Eyes, vision – light sensitivity, increased (photophobia)
Gait – ataxic
Head – pain (headache)
Heart rate – slow (bradycardia)
Mentation – confused
Mentation – delirium
Mentation – sleepy (somnolence)
Mentation – weakness (malaise)
Mood – labile
Mood – lethargic
Mood – restless, irritable
Muscles, up/low unilat – weakness (hemiparesis) [1]
Muscles – pain (myalgia)
Muscles – paralysis
Nausea
Neck, posterior – pain
Neck, posterior – stiff (meningismus)
Seizures
Sign: Brudzinski's
Sign: Kernig's

Speech – disturbed (dysphasia)
Sweating – increased (hyperhydrosis)
Temperature, body – elevated (fever)
Urination, spontaneous control – loss (urinary incontinence)
Vomiting

Laboratory

Blood sodium – decreased [2]
CSF glucose – decreased [4]
CSF protein – increased
CSF pressure – increased
CSF WBC – increased [4]

Imaging

Computed tomography – brain [3]
Magnetic resonance imaging – brain [3]

Other Tests

EEG – NS changes

Notes

[1]   Sudden onset; hemiparesis with tendon reflex asymmetry and positive
      Babinski sign
[2]   Inappropriate antidiuretic hormone secretion
[3]   For focal areas of hemorrhage or inflammation
[4]   Bacterial etiology

http://www.argus1.com/?meningencephcomp

Updates

_____
_____
_____
_____
_____
_____
_____
_____
_____
_____
_____

Myocarditis

Clinical Guide **Primary Conditions**
Arsine poisoning
Avian influenza
Chickenpox
Dengue
Ebola hemorrhagic fever
Infectious nucleosis
Influenza
Lassa fever
Legionellosis
Leptospirosis
Lyme disease
Lymphocytic choriomeningitis
Marburg hemorrhagic fever
Meningococcemia
Mumps
Psittacosis
Q fever
Rocky Mountain spotted fever
Rubeola
Shigellosis
Smallpox
Trichinellosis
Typhus – scrub
West Nile fever
Yersiniosis

Signs/Symptoms [7]
Breathing – diff, effort (effort dyspnea) [8]
Breathing – diff, reclining flat (orthopnea) [8]
Breathing – diff, rest (rest dyspnea) [8]

Chest, ant – pain, nonpleuritic rest
Chest, ant – pain, pleuritic [2]
Chest, ant – palpitations
Chest – rales [8]
Cough – acute NS [3]
Extremities, lower bilat – edema
Fatigue
Heart, LV apex – murmur, systolic [6, 8]
Heart – friction rub
Heart rate – rapid (tachycardia) [4]
Heart rhythm – irregular [5]
Heart sound S1 – soft
Heart sound – S3 LV [8]
Joints – pain (arthralgia) [3]
Mentation – weakness (malaise)
Muscles – pain (myalgia)
Temperature, body – elevated (fever)
Urine – decreased (oliguria) [8]

Laboratory

Blood troponin I – increased
Blood troponin T – increased
Other cardiac enzymes – increased

ECG

Dysrhythmias, atrial
Dysrhythmias, conduction
Dysrhythmias, ventricular
Q wave – abnormal [1]
ST-T wave – nonspecific abnormality

Imaging

Heart, general – enlarged [8]
Lungs, vasculature – congested [8]

Other Tests

Myocardial biopsy

Notes

[1]   Esp Coxsackievirus infection
[2]   Pericardial involvement

[3]   Due to prior or concurrent infection
[4]   Disproportionate to fever
[5]   Ventricular premature beats, atrial premature beats, atrial arrhythmias, conduction abnormalities all may occur
[6]   Transient
[7]   Often asymptomatic
[8]   With left ventricular dysfunction

http://www.argus1.com/?myocarditis

Updates

_____
_____
_____
_____
_____
_____
_____
_____
_____
_____
_____
_____
_____
_____
_____
_____
_____
_____
_____

Noncardiac Pulmonary Edema

Clinical Guide Primary Conditions

Ammonia poisoning
Arsine poisoning
Barium poisoning
Benzene poisoning
Bromine poisoning
Carbon monoxide poisoning
Chlorine poisoning
Cholera
Cyanide poisoning
Ethylene glycol poisoning
Hantavirus pulmonary syndrome
Hemorrhagic fever with renal syndrome
Lewisite poisoning
Malaria
Mercury poisoning
Methyl bromide poisoning
Methyl isocyanate poisoning
Opioid poisoning
Osmium tetroxide poisoning
Phosgene poisoning
Phosphine poisoning
Ricin poisoning
Rocky Mountain spotted fever
Smallpox
Sulfuryl fluoride poisoning
Sulfur mustard poisoning

Signs/Symptoms

Breathing – diff, acute (acute dyspnea)
Breathing – diff, effort (effort dyspnea)

Breathing – diff, rest (rest dyspnea)
Breathing – rapid (tachypnea)
Breath sounds – crackling (rales)
Cough – acute nonspecific
Fatigue
Heart rate – rapid (tachycardia)
Mood – anxious
Skin color – blue (cyanosis)

Laboratory

Blood, arterial pCO_2 – decreased
Blood, arterial pH – increased (alkalosis)
Blood, arterial pO_2 – decreased (hypoxia)

Imaging

Lungs, parenchyma – edema

Other Tests

NS

http://www.argus1.com/?puledema

Updates

_____
_____
_____
_____
_____
_____
_____
_____
_____
_____
_____
_____
_____
_____
_____
_____

Orchitis

Clinical Guide Primary Conditions
Brucellosis
Ebola hemorrhagic fever
Glanders
Infectious mononucleosis
Lassa fever
Lymphocytic choriomeningitis
Marburg hemorrhagic fever
Mumps
Rubella
Smallpox

Signs/Symptoms
Lymph nodes, inguinal – enlarged
Lymph nodes, inguinal – tender
Pelvis, groin – swelling
Penis, ejaculation – pain
Penis, intercourse – pain
Penis, semen – blood (hematospermia)
Penis – discharge
Prostate – enlarged
Prostate – tender
Scrotum – swollen
Temperature, body – elevated (fever)
Testicles – pain/heaviness
Testicles – swelling
Testicles – tender
Urination – pain

Imaging
Doppler ultrasound testicle
Nuclear medicine scan testicle

http://www.argus1.com/?orchitis

Updates

_____

_____

_____

_____

_____

_____

_____

_____

_____

_____

_____

_____

_____

_____

_____

_____

_____

_____

_____

_____

Osteomyelitis

Clinical Guide Primary Conditions
Brucellosis
Chickenpox
Glanders
Meningococcemia
Q fever
Salmonellosis
Smallpox
Streptococcal pharyngitis
Tularemia

Signs/Symptoms
Bone, local – pain
Bone, local – tender
Bone, overlying skin – red
Bone, overlying soft tissue – swelling
Chills
Mentation – weakness (malaise)
Nausea
Sweating – increased (hyperhydrosis)
Temperature, body – elevated (fever)

Laboratory
Blood alkaline phosphatase – increased
Blood culture – positive [1]
Blood WBC – increased (leukocytosis) [1]

Imaging [2]
Bone changes may be diagnostic

Other Tests
Bone biopsy/culture

Notes
[1] Depends on causative organism
[2] May be diagnostic and findings vary according to agent and duration of infection

http://www.argus1.com/?osteomyelitis

Updates

_____
_____
_____
_____
_____
_____
_____
_____
_____
_____
_____
_____
_____
_____
_____
_____
_____
_____
_____
_____

Pancreatitis

Clinical Guide Primary Conditions

Cryptosporidiosis
Ebola hemorrhagic fever
Infectious mononucleosis
Legionellosis
Marburg hemorrhagic fever
Mumps
Organophosphate poisoning
Psittacosis
Typhoid fever
West Nile fever

Signs/Symptoms

Abdomen – pain
Abdomen – tender
Chills
Mood – anxious
Muscles – weak
Nausea
Skin color – yellow (jaundice) [1]
Stools – fatty
Sweating – increased (hyperhydrosis)
Temperature, body – elevated (fever)
Weight – loss
Vomiting

Laboratory

Blood amylase – increased
Blood bilirubin – increased [1]
Blood calcium – decreased
Blood glucose – increased

Blood lipase – increased
Blood SGOT – increased
Blood urea nitrogen – increased
Blood WBC – increased (leukocytosis)

Imaging
Abdominal ultrasound
Abdominal CT

Note
[1]   Usually mild elevation

http://www.argus1.com/?pancreatitis

Updates

_____
_____
_____
_____
_____
_____
_____
_____
_____
_____
_____
_____
_____
_____
_____
_____
_____
_____
_____
_____
_____

Pericarditis

Note: often occurs concurrently with myocarditis.

Clinical Guide Primary Conditions

Avian influenza
Influenza
Infectious mononucleosis
Lassa fever
Legionellosis
Leptospirosis
Listeriosis
Lyme disease
Meningococcemia
Psittacosis
Q fever
Salmonellosis
Sulfuryl fluoride poisoning
Tularemia
Typhoid fever

Signs/Symptoms

Abdomen, epigastrium – pain
Breathing – difficult, rest (rest dyspnea)
Chest – pain, left supraclavicular
Chest – pain, nonpleuritic [1]
Chest – pain, pleuritic [1]
Consciousness – loss, sudden NS (syncope)
Cough – acute nonspecific
Fatigue
Heart, lower LSB – friction rub
Heart, mid LSB – friction rub
Hiccups

Swallowing – difficult (dysphagia)
Temperature, body – elevated (fever)

Laboratory

Blood, troponin I – increased [2]
Blood, troponin T – increased [2]

ECG

Dysrhythmias, atrial
PR segment – depressed
ST segment – elevated
T wave – inversion, abnormal
Voltage, general – decreased

Imaging

Echocardiogram – pericardial fluid [3]

Other Tests

Pericardiocentesis

Notes

[1]   Relieved by sitting up
[2]   Due to concurrent myocarditis
[3]   Ranges from minimal to large amount

http://www.argus1.com/?secpericard

Updates

_____
_____
_____
_____
_____
_____
_____
_____
_____
_____
_____

Pneumonia

Note: pneumonia can occur due to infection by the primary agent or secondarily due to damage and compromize of pulmonary tissue to defense against outside bacteria.

Clinical Guide Primary Conditions

Ammonia poisoning
Avian influenza
Botulism
Brucellosis
Chickenpox
Chlorine poisoning
Cholera
Glanders
Infectious mononucleosis
Influenza
Listeriosis
Methyl bromide poisoning
Methyl isocyanate poisoning
Omsk hemorrhagic fever
Osmium tetroxide poisoning
Pertussis
Radiation poisoning
Rocky Mountain spotted fever
Rubeola
Smallpox
Streptococcal pharyngitis
Sulfur mustard poisoning
Trichinellosis
Tularemia
Typhus – epidemic
Typhus – scrub
Yellow fever

Signs/Symptoms

Appetite – decreased (anorexia)
Breathing, rest – difficult (rest dyspnea)
Breathing – rapid (tachypnea)
Breath sounds, local – bronchial
Breath sounds, local – coarse (rhonchi, local)
Breath sounds, local – crackling (rales, local)
Breath sounds, local – decreased
Chest, ant – pain, pleuritic
Chest, lat – pain, pleuritic
Chest, local – percussion dullness
Chest, post – pain, pleuritic
Chest – fremitus, vocal
Chest – friction rub, pleural
Chest – pectoriloquy, local
Chills
Cough – acute NS
Cough – productive
Fatigue
Head – pain (headache)
Mentation – confused [1]
Nausea
Sputum – blood (hemoptysis)
Sputum – purulent
Sweating – increased (hyperhydrosis)
Temperature, body – elevated (fever)
Vomiting

Laboratory

Blood culture
Blood WBC – increased (leukocytosis)
Pleural fluid bacterial stain
Pleural fluid culture
Sputum stain
Sputum WBC

Imaging

Chest – infiltrates and other abnormalities depending on type and
duration

Note
[1]   Esp older persons

http://www.argus1.com/?secpneumonia

Updates

_____
_____
_____
_____
_____
_____
_____
_____
_____
_____
_____
_____
_____
_____
_____
_____
_____
_____
_____
_____

Renal Failure

Note: Renal failure can be caused by direct tissue damage from the causative agent or by sufficiently severe and prolonged hypotension, especially when prior renal disease is present.

Clinical Guide Primary Conditions

Arsenic poisoning
Arsine poisoning
Barium poisoning
Benzene poisoning
Cholera
Colchicine poisoning
Crimean-Congo hemorrhagic fever
Ebola hemorrhagic fever
E coli 0157:H7
Ethylene glycol poisoning
Leptospirosis
Lewisite poisoning
Malaria
Marburg hemorrhagic fever
Meningococcemia
Methyl bromide poisoning
Phosgene poisoning
Phosphine poisoning
Radiation poisoning
Rocky Mountain spotted fever
Sulfuryl fluoride poisoning
Tetrodotoxin poisoning
Trichothecene poisoning
Typhus – epidemic
Typhus – murine
Typhus – scrub
Yellow fever

Signs/Symptoms
Abdomen, flank – pain
Appetite – reduced (anorexia)
Arterial press – elevated
Bleeding – easy
Body, general – edema (anasarca)
Bowel movements, stool – blood or black (hematochezia) (melena)
Consciousness – loss, prolonged (coma)
Extremities, lower bilat – edema
Extremities – tremors
Fatigue
Hiccups
Mentation – concentration impaired
Mentation – confused
Mentation – delirium
Mentation – hallucinations
Mentation – sleepiness (somnolence)
Mentation – nonspecific changes
Mood – labile
Mood – lethargic
Mood – restless/irritable
Muscles – movement, slow/sluggish
Nausea
Nose – blood (epistaxis)
Seizures
Sense of taste – metallic
Skin – bruising, easy
Urination – nighttime (nocturia)
Urine – absent (anuria)
Urine – reduced (oliguria)
Vomiting

Laboratory
Blood arterial pH – decreased (acidosis)
Blood creatinine – increased
Blood creatinine clearance – decreased
Blood potassium – increased
Blood urea nitrogen – increased
Urine – abnormal per underlying cause

ECG

NS abnormalities
T wave – peaked [1]

Imaging

Lower urinary tract [2]
Renal

Other Tests

Cystoscopy [2]

Notes

[1] Hyperkalemia
[2] For obstructive lesions

http://www.argus1.com/?acuterenal

Updates

_____
_____
_____
_____
_____
_____
_____
_____
_____
_____
_____
_____
_____
_____
_____
_____
_____
_____
_____
_____
_____

Respiratory Failure

Note: respiratory failure is more likely to occur in the presence of prior lung disease and settings of abnormal tissue oxygen exchange, such as anemia.

Clinical Guide Primary Conditions

Anthrax
Arsenic poisoning
Benzene poisoning
Botulism
Chlorine poisoning
Colchicine poisoning
Cyanide poisoning
Hantavirus pulmonary syndrome
Leptospirosis
Lewisite poisoning
Malaria
Meningococcemia
Mercury poisoning
Methyl bromide poisoning
Nicotine poisoning
Organophosphate poisoning
Phosgene poisoning
Psittacosis
Ricin poisoning
Rocky Mountain spotted fever
Sarin poisoning
SARS
Sodium monofluoroacetate poisoning
Strychnine poisoning
Sulfuryl fluoride poisoning
Tabun poisoning
Tetrodotoxin poisoning
Thallium poisoning
Trichinellosis
Trichothecene poisoning

Tularemia
Typhus – murine
Western equine encephalitis
West Nile fever

Signs/Symptoms

Breathing – diff, acute (acute dyspnea)
Breathing – diff, rest (rest dyspnea)
Breathing – rapid (tachypnea)
Consciousness – altered
Fatigue
Head – pain (headache)
Heart rate – rapid (tachycardia)
Mentation – concentration impaired
Mentation – confused
Mentation – sleepiness (somnolence)
Mood – anxious
Mood – depressed
Seizures
Skin color – blue (cyanosis)

Laboratory

Blood arterial pO_2 – decreased (hypoxia)
Blood arterial pCO_2 – increased
Blood arterial pH – decreased (acidosis)

Imaging

Chest/lung findings vary according to pulmonary etiology and may be normal if cause is extra-pulmonary, i.e., paralysis of chest muscles

http://www.argus1.com/?respfailure

Updates

_____
_____
_____
_____
_____
_____
_____

Rhabdomyolysis

Clinical Guide Primary Conditions

Avian influenza
Barium poisoning
Carbon monoxide poisoning
Colchicine poisoning
Cyanide poisoning
Influenza
Leptospirosis
Listeriosis
Tularemia

Signs/Symptoms

Fatigue
Joints, gen – pain (arthralgia)
Muscles – pain (myalgia)
Muscles – stiff
Muscles – tender
Muscles – weak
Seizures
Urine – dark
Weight – gain

Laboratory

Blood creatine phosphokinase (CPK) – increased
Blood creatinine – increased
Blood myoglobin – increased
Blood potassium – increased [2]
Urine hemoglobin – present (hemoglobinuria) [1]
Urine myoglobin – present

Notes

[1]   No RBCS on microscopic exam

[2]   May be very high

http://www.argus1.com/?rhabdo

Updates

_____

_____

_____

_____

_____

_____

_____

_____

_____

_____

_____

_____

_____

_____

_____

_____

_____

_____

_____

_____

Thrombocytopenia

Clinical Guide Primary Conditions

Brucellosis
E coli 0157:H7 [3]
Chickenpox
Colchicine poisoning
Meningococcemia
Radiation poisoning
Psittacosis
Rubella

Signs/Symptoms [1]

Bleeding, gen – minimal trauma/spontaneous
Skin – ecchymoses
Skin – rash, petechiae
Skin – rash, purpura

Laboratory [1]

Blood, platelets – decreased (thrombocytopenia)

Note

[1]   PT and PTT normal

http://www.argus1.com/?thrombocyto

Updates

_____
_____
_____
_____
_____

DIFFERENTIAL DIAGNOSIS BY SYSTEM

Note: *The page numbers following each diagnosis refer the reader to the discussion in the text.*

Cardiovascular

Coagulation

Gastrointestinal

Hematopoietic/Immune

Liver/Biliary Tract/Pancreas

Nervous

Optic

Oropharynx

Renal/Genitourinary

Respiratory – Lower

Respiratory – Upper

Skin

SYMBOLS AND ABBREVIATIONS

Abbreviations

ADH	Antidiuretic hormone
AIDS	Autoimmune deficiency syndrome
ANT	Anterior
ART	Arterial
AV	Atrioventricular
BLOOD	Blood or bleeding
BNP	B-type natriuretic peptide
BP	Blood pressure
BSL	Biosafety level
CDC	Centers for Disease Control
CNS	Central nervous system
COPD	Chronic obstructive pulmonary disease
CSF	Cerebrospinal fluid
CT	Computed or computerized tomography
DIC	Disseminated intravasculer coagulation
DIFF	Difficult
EM	Electron microscopy
EMG	Electromyogram
ELISA	Enzyme-Linked ImmunoSorbent Assay
ESP	Especially
GEN	General
GI	Gastrointestinal
HBO	Hyperbaric oxygenation
HCT	Hematocrit
HGB	Hemoglobin
IV	Intravenous
LAT	Lateral
LDH	Lactic dehydrogenase
LE	Lower extremity
LSB	Left sternal border
LSD	Lysergic acid diethylamide

LUQ	Left upper quadrant
LV	Left Ventricle
MIP	Metacarpal interphalangeal
NA	Not applicable
ND	Not determined; inadequate evidence or data
NS	Non-specific
PIP	Proximal interphalangeal
POST	Posterior
PRESS	Pressure
PT	Prothrombin time
PTT	Partial thromboplastin time
RBC	Red blood cells
RV	Right ventricle
S3	Third heart sound
S4	Fourth heart sound
SCBA	Self contained breathing apparatus
SE	Southeast
TEMP	Temperature
UE	Upper extremity
USA	United States of America
WBC	White blood cells
WHO	World Health Organization
IE	Such as, for example
ECG	Electrocardiogram

Symbols

☠ Relates to fatality
▲ Warning, caution, danger▲
[ ] Indicates "Note" at end of disease, with number in brackets
( ) Medical term or clarifying word
? Uncertain fact or status
< Less than
> Greater than
/ And, or
+ Positive for